Not Just Sadness

The silence needs to be heard!

Dr. Sloka

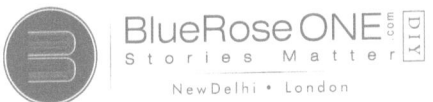

BLUEROSE PUBLISHERS
India | U.K.

Copyright © Dr. Sloka 2024

All rights reserved by author. No part of this publication may be reproduced, stored in a retrieval system or transmitted in any form or by any means, electronic, mechanical, photocopying, recording or otherwise, without the prior permission of the author. Although every precaution has been taken to verify the accuracy of the information contained herein, the publisher assume no responsibility for any errors or omissions. No liability is assumed for damages that may result from the use of information contained within.

BlueRose Publishers takes no responsibility for any damages, losses, or liabilities that may arise from the use or misuse of the information, products, or services provided in this publication.

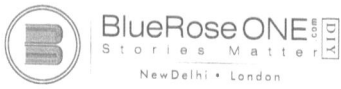

For permissions requests or inquiries regarding this publication, please contact:

BLUEROSE PUBLISHERS
www.BlueRoseONE.com
info@bluerosepublishers.com
+91 8882 898 898
+4407342408967

ISBN: 978-93-6261-448-3

First Edition: May 2024

To all those fighting the silent battle

May your silence be heard in the darkest moments of your journey!

Easy to die in life
But it's not what life is meant for
Ease your life with dyes of your own thoughts
There's no greater joy than sharing your untold story of suffering inside you

---

Dr. Sloka

The benefits of this book written by an author that has a clear understanding of the impact that Depression has on an individual is detrimental in aiding those who struggle to find a balance in life. It gives the reader comfort in knowing that they are not alone in their struggles and there is light at the end of the tunnel.

A route to a brighter future

Judy Alloway
Mental Health First Aider
United Kingdom

This book shows how much we all at times struggle with depression and mental health. The author shows empathy, compassion and understanding of how people suffering with depression battle their own demons on the darker days of the illness

Deborah Rutter
Manager, In-Patients
NHS, United Kingdom

This book is nothing like a friend in need, it is like a ray of hope in the darkness of depression. Depression is like a war which results in mental destruction if not supported properly and this book serves as the Gita before the war.

Vamshi Gattu
Peer Supporter
United Kingdom

ABOUT THE AUTHOR

Dr. Sloka, a pen name for Dr. Sukesh Krishna Chaitanya Loka, holds a doctors degree in Pharmacology and Therapeutics and a Master's degree in Clinical Psychology. His credentials also include certification as a psychometrics testing professional, a skill that enables him to delve deeper into understanding human attitudes, personalities, and behaviours. He's the author of the book "**The Unspoken Thoughts**"; a collection of his poems in various styles. While writing this book, Dr. Sloka was serving at an esteemed Mental Health Trust of the NHS in the United Kingdom where he was also the Health and Well-being champion.

He was trained in Mindfulness Based Cognitive Therapy (MBCT) by the TEWV NHS foundation trust, and Suicide Prevention by the "If u care share" foundation in the United Kingdom. He was also trained in Cognitive Behavioural Therapy (CBT), self-compassion, HIV Counselling, arts therapy, and psychosexual therapy. His broad knowledge base and dedication to these disciplines enable him to provide holistic and compassionate care to his clients.

Dr. Sloka has worked with clients facing an array of mental health challenges, including anxiety, depression, panic attacks, and obsessive-compulsive disorder (OCD), stress, relationship difficulties, and sexual issues and many others. His compassionate and comprehensive approach to therapy has allowed him to assist individuals in their journeys toward mental well-being.

In addition to his clinical work, his research in the realm of mental health is both extensive and varied. Notably, he has delved into the impact of managerial personalities on the job satisfaction of employees in the workplace. This exploration illustrates his commitment to fostering healthier and more harmonious work environments. Dr. Sloka has also presented numerous lectures on the subject of mental health, further contributing to the awareness on mental well-being.

He can be contacted on his e-mail address sukeshloka@gmail.com or his Facebook and Instagram handle ***@SukeshKrishnaChaitanyaLoka***, should anyone need his support/guidance.

ACKNOWLEDGEMENT

"There can be no rainbow without a cloud and a storm."
- John J. Vincent

You never know the value of empathy until you've experienced the despair and so this wonderful resource of **"Not Just Sadness; the silence needs to be heard"** wouldn't have taken birth if I've never had encountered both the despair and the empathy.

I extend my heartfelt gratitude to the following individuals whose unwavering support and empathy have been instrumental in my life.

Lesley Geddes, the Director of the Healthcare academics at the Northumbria University, United Kingdom. Your kindness and unconditional support after a traumatic event in my life were a guiding light. Your in-person assistance and academic encouragement were invaluable.

Claire Slaughter, manager at the North East Urgent Care Services, your help in offering flexibility in working patterns, regular check-ins, and the use of non-stigmatizing language have made a significant impact.

Judy Alloway, your love and kindness, treating me like your son, warmed my heart during challenging times. Your presence was a comforting beacon and your support has not gone unnoticed.

To my pillars of strength, **Vamshi** and **Vaishnavi**, you have been like siblings from other mothers, offering unwavering support during times of crisis & appreciate you knowing the importance of mental health.

Deborah Rutter, my superior, thank you for helping me strike a balance between work and life. Your understanding was a breath of fresh air.

To **Rakesh, Sandeep**, friends since the childhood and the friends, in the USA, UK, Canada, and India, **Prasad** in Germany, **Srikanth** in the Australia; your love, support, and strong bond have been instrumental. Your dismissal comments were the catalyst that reminded me that spreading awareness on mental health begins within our own networks.

To **Ashok and Shekar,** who have been with me offering their moral support at all the needed times and showed how 'someone being there for me' can be highly remarkable.

To **Anusha**, you've been a companion in distress for more than a decade, a friend whom I fear no loss. Your presence has been a constant source of solace. We're not just friends, but partners in mental suffering too: P

To **Swetha**, your support during the times of my suffering was so therapeutic!

To my family, my parents **Sukanya and Venkatesh**, my sister and brother-in-law **Sudheshna &Varun**, you've been unwavering in your love, kindness, and support through every adversity and of course, you're no exception to becoming aware on breaking stereotypes and stigma

To my wife, **Rupali**, your maturity, understanding, love, and support have been my bedrock. Your awareness of the importance of mental health is deeply appreciated. I'm proud of you and lucky to have you as my partner.

To, my father-in-law **Srinivas**, your attention and care for a family member suffering from depression, and attitude towards mental health is so heart-touching

To my four-legged friend, **Snufy**, more than a pet, you've offered unconditional love. You're now in a place of eternal joy, and your presence remains irreplaceable.

Last but certainly not least, I extend my appreciation to all the people in my life, including relatives, flatmates, and friends, colleagues, patients who either showed empathy, kindness, or even passed judgmental or dismissal comments. It is through these experiences that I found resilience and strength. Your collective support and understanding have been instrumental in the creation of this guide. Thank you for being a part of this journey.

And, finally! How can I forget you the gorgeous reader, thank you very much for picking this valuable resource and taking time out to read this. Happy reading!

- *Dr. Sloka*

WHO IS THIS GUIDE FOR?

If you're reading this page to know who this guide is for, it is undoubtedly for you. Whether you suffered depression or any any other mental illness in silence, and looking for a support or have witnessed someone suffering the mental problems and didn't know how to support them, then this book, "**Not Just Sadness; the silence needs to be heard**", becomes a wonderful tool to increase your awareness about the most challenging and not much spoken mental health illness, depression, to challenge stigma and expand your learning on how to offer support and foster encouragement to your loved ones suffering from depression and helping them in the part of their recovery journey.

It is also intended for psychologists, psychology students, counsellors, and all other mental health professionals seeking a comprehensive understanding of depression and practical guidance on how to support their clients actively break the stigma and stereotypes associated with it.

Family members, friends, and loved ones can become more informed, empathetic allies in the battle against depression, ultimately fostering a stronger support system.

Ultimately, this book is a powerful tool for anyone seeking to develop a comprehensive knowledge of depression and to become a mental health advocate within their own network. It encourages a holistic approach to mental health, emphasizing awareness, compassion, and active support for those facing depression.

Note: The book is to create an awareness about depression, and it's important to note that the information provided is not a substitute for professional medical advice. If you or anyone you know is struggling with mental health issues, please consult a doctor.

PREFACE

Have you ever encountered the comments like, "you should be strong in life, why are you sad all the time as if you lost something"?, "what are you short of in life- you're educated, earning well, you've got parents, a good job, a fancy car, and a house. What makes you feel depressed yet?" And thought "it's as if you've personally experienced everything in my life with the way you're commenting". Can you relate?

In the quiet shadows of our homes, behind closed doors and fake smiles, millions of individuals fight with a silent issue: depression. Hearing those comments can be more distressing than the actual pain and suffering.

"Not Just Sadness; the silence needs to be heard" was born out of hearing those comments and a feeling "I wish my family, friends, and relatives knew what mental health struggles are and how to offer support". At first, I believed that I was the only one who felt this way but, during my practice of counseling and therapy with patients, I realized a lot many people suffering depression are feeling the same way that their journey would have been better if their families had a good understanding of what they're suffering. It is then clear that "I am not alone and neither you're". We all need support and we deserve it.

Depression is a battle that affects people from all walks of life. Yet, despite its prevalence, depression remains covered in stigma and misunderstanding. As you read through the pages, I am sure you'll shed your preconceived notions and prejudices. I invite you to step into the shoes of those who walk the path of depression every day.

In these pages, I'll tell you the complexities of depression, from its causes to its myriad manifestations. You'll learn practical strategies for offering support, for nurturing the bonds that tie families together even when faced with the most formidable of challenges. **You'll find stories of resilience and hope, from individuals who have braved the darkest storms and emerged stronger.**

My aim is clear: to make everyone understand that every individual's journey with depression is unique, and there is no one-size-fits-all solution. Shatter the walls of silence of depression and it is now time to replace ignorance with knowledge, judgment with compassion, and isolation with community. The process begins within these pages, but it extends far beyond them. It extends into our homes, our hearts, and our actions. More than anything, it begins with ourselves.

Join me on this journey as I'd explore the profound impact of depression on individuals and their families, seek to understand its origins and manifestations, and equip ourselves with the tools needed to foster resilience, compassion, and hope.

Yes, together, we can break the stigma. We can learn, and understand. Together, we can make a difference. Together, we can create a mentally healthy world.

With heartfelt dedication.

Dr. Sloka

WHAT'S INSIDE ?

1. Understanding Depression and The Stigma 1

    1.1 D for DEPRESSION, lets define it! 2
    1.2 How common is depression? 3
    1.3 The complex nature of depression............................. 4
        1.3.1. Types of Depression.. 4
        1.3.2 Common Symptoms of Depression.................... 6
        1.3.3 Is Depression the same in everyone? 6
    1.4 Stigma and Depression 8
    1.5 Myths and facts around Depression 11
    1.6 How to challenge misconceptions? 13

2. The Depth Of Depression 16

    2.1 Recognizing The Signs and Symptoms of
        Depression..16
        2.1.1 Common Emotional Symptoms.........................16
        2.1.2 Behavioral Signs of Depression 17
        2.1.3 Physical Symptoms to Watch For......................19
    2.2 Red Flags to Look for- warning signs for suicide..... 20
    2.3 Sadness and Depression- are they both same? 21
    2.4 What causes Depression? 22
        2.4.1 Biological Factors: Genetic Predisposition...... 22
        2.4.2 Environmental Factors: Early Life
            Experiences 24
        2.4.3 Psychosocial factors.. 25
    2.5 The Common Triggers 25
        2.5.1 The Role of Life Transitions 25
        2.5.2 Relationship Struggles and Loss...................... 27

2.5.3 Substance Abuse and Its Connection to
Depression 28
2.5.4 Co-occurring Mental Health Disorders 29

3. Pathways to Healing 31

3.1 The Mental Health Specialists 31
3.2 The Role of Mental Health Team 34
3.3 The Process of Diagnosis 37
3.4 Treatment Modalities.. 39
    3.4.1 Psychotherapy (Talk Therapy)..........................40
    3.4.2 Drug Therapy 41
    3.4.3 Lifestyle Changes and Behavioral
         Interventions (Instant mood up lifters)..........45
3.5 But! What stops us?... 48
    3.5.1 Stigma as a Barrier to Seeking Help 48
    3.5.2 Financial and Access Barriers 51
    3.5.3 Medication Concerns and Side Effects 52
3.6 Family, the First Support Group 54
    3.6.1 Supporting Treatment Adherence..................... 54
    3.6.2 Communicating with Healthcare Providers 56
3.7 Dealing with CRISIS SITUATIONS............................. 58
    3.7.1 Alert Signs 58
    3.7.2 What to Do in an Emergency?........................... 59

4. Extend Love, End Stigma 62

4.1 E- Empathetic Communication 62
    4.1.1 The Power of Listening 63
    4.1.2 Effective Conversation Strategies-
         What to say?... 63
    4.1.3 Avoiding Common Pitfalls in Communication-
         what not to say? 65
4.2 E- Emotional Support and Encouragement 67
4.3 E- Engaging 68

4.4 E- Educate family and beyond 71

5. Recovery 75
5.1 The Real Story of Hope and Resilience 75
5.2 The Reflection 79
5.3 Navigating Setbacks and Challenges 80
5.4 A Future Filled with Hope 82

Final Words 84
References 86

1. UNDERSTANDING DEPRESSION AND THE STIGMA

"Behind every untold story and the unheard history,
are the tears hidden in smiles,
Not every pain is cried out loud, some sufferings are silent" -Dr. Sloka

Imagine a world where we openly talk about our emotions, where seeking help for mental health is as natural as visiting a doctor for a physical ailment. In such a world, understanding and supporting loved ones dealing with depression wouldn't be a mystery or a challenge wrapped in stigma. We'd all know how to reach out, how to offer a listening ear, and how to help.

But, unfortunately, we're not there yet. Depression remains a shadowy figure in our society. It's the quiet struggle that many suffer behind the closed doors, sometimes feeling too ashamed or too misunderstood to seek the help they need. It's a silent battle within our own minds.

In this first part of the book, let's take a look at what depression is, breaking it down into simpler terms, free from academic jargon. I'll talk about what depression really is, and how it affects those who experience it. We'll also delve into the uncomfortable truth that, in many cases, the real challenge isn't just dealing with depression but also the stigma that surrounds it.

1.1 D for DEPRESSION, lets define it!

We all know that life is a complex and ever-changing journey filled with different moments of joy, sorrow, triumph, and struggle. We all experience our ups and downs, navigating the ebb and flow of emotions. But for some, this natural rhythm can become a storm that never seems to pass – a relentless, overwhelming weight that casts a long shadow on everyday life affecting relationships, personal, professional, social and other walks of life. This is the essence of depression.

Depression is more than just feeling sad or having a bad day. According to *Diagnostic and Statistical Manual of Mental Disorders-* 5 (DSM-5), depression is a serious and pervasive mental health illness or a mood disorder causing persistent feelings of sadness, and loss of interest. It doesn't discriminate by age, gender, or background, and it can affect anyone – from the teenager struggling to find their place in the world to the seasoned adult juggling life's demands.

When someone is depressed, it's not easy for them to enjoy the things they used to love. They might lose interest in hobbies, friends, and even their own well-being. Even getting out of bed in the morning can feel like an enormous task.

Depression can also mess with a person's thinking. It fills their mind with negative thoughts, self-doubt, and a sense of hopelessness. It's like having a mean voice inside their head that constantly tells them they're not good enough and keeps poking them from inside.

This condition isn't a sign of weakness or a choice but a **real illness** that affects the brain and emotions and thereby various aspects of the everyday life. And the good news is, just like with any other illness, there are ways to treat and manage it but the key here is to understand the depression as this is the first step in helping someone you care about find their way back to a brighter, happier life.

1.2 How common is depression?

Know what! Depression is more common than you might think. It's not something that only a few people experience or people who lost something would need to experience. In fact, it's one of the most widespread mental health challenges in the world. Surprising right! It is estimated that about 5% of population in the world suffer from depression and more than 700,000 people die due to suicide every year making suicide the fourth highest cause of death.

Remember the famous Indian celebrity Sushant Singh Rajput's case? There are a several cases in which people lost their lives by suicide. Depression affects 1 in 10 people.

If you look around, you'll realize that you probably know someone who has gone through depression, even if they haven't talked about it. That's because millions of people from all walks of life, regardless of age, gender, or background, have faced depression at some point in their lives.

It's like a silent epidemic that affects our friends, family, colleagues, and even ourselves. This prevalence emphasizes the importance of understanding and addressing depression – not as something rare, but as something that touches us all in some way.

Depression has the power to alter the very fabric of an individual's existence, leading to emotional turmoil, impaired work life balance, emotional exhaustion, and financial burden and affecting the overall quality of life.

1.3 The complex nature of depression

Depression is not a one-size-fits-all condition. It's a complex and multifaceted experience that varies from person to person. Imagine it as a puzzle with many pieces, each representing different aspects of this mental health challenge. As we explore the complexity of depression, we'll uncover several important dimensions: such as the various types of depression, the commonest symptoms (a detailed information is in the section 2), and the variability of the depression's expression.

1.3.1. Types of Depression

Depression comes in various forms, and understanding these types can help individuals and their healthcare providers determine the most appropriate treatment. Here are some of the most common types of depression:

Type of depression	Characteristics
Major Depressive Disorder (MDD):	It involves a persistent low mood, loss of interest or pleasure in most activities, and other symptoms that interfere with daily life. MDD often includes feelings of hopelessness and worthlessness
Persistent Depressive Disorder (Dysthymia)	Dysthymia is a milder, but more chronic form of depression. It involves long-lasting symptoms that may not be as severe as MDD but can still significantly affect a person's life
Bipolar Disorder	Formerly known as manic depression, bipolar disorder involves cycling between periods of depression and periods of mania or hypomania (elevated mood, increased energy, and impulsivity). There are different types of bipolar disorder, such as Bipolar I and Bipolar II, depending on the severity of the manic episodes
Seasonal Affective	SAD is a type of depression that tends to occur at specific times of the year, most commonly in the fall and winter when

Disorder (SAD)	there's less natural sunlight. Symptoms typically improve in the spring and summer
Psychotic Depression	In this type of depression, individuals experience severe depression along with psychotic symptoms, such as delusions or hallucinations. It's essential to treat both the depressive and psychotic symptoms
Peripartum Depression	It was formerly called postpartum depression and occurs in some women either during or after giving birth. It involves feelings of extreme sadness, anxiety, and exhaustion that can interfere with their ability to care for themselves and their new born
Premenstrual Dysphoric Disorder (PMDD)	PMDD is a severe form of premenstrual syndrome (PMS) characterized by significant mood disturbances in the luteal phase of the menstrual cycle
Atypical Depression	Atypical depression is a subtype of major depressive disorder with specific features such as an improved mood in response to positive events, excessive sleep, increased appetite, and a heavy sensation in the limbs.
Cyclothymic Disorder	Cyclothymia is a milder form of bipolar disorder, characterized by chronic mood disturbances, but not as severe as in bipolar I or II.
Situational Depression	Also known as adjustment disorder with depressed mood, this type of depression is usually triggered by a specific life event, such as a job loss, divorce, or loss of a loved one
Melancholic depression	Severe form of depression accompanied by agitation, extreme weight loss, no pleasure, grief

Other types may also include treatment resistant depression, recurrent brief depression, substance induced mood disorders, mood disorders due to physical illness.

1.3.2 Common Symptoms of Depression

Depression can manifest in a variety of ways, and people experience a combination of symptoms to varying degrees of severity and section 2 has more details about the symptoms but the common symptoms of depression are

- Persistent Sadness
- Loss of Interest or Pleasure
- Changes in Sleep Patterns
- Fatigue and Low Energy
- Changes in Appetite and Weight
- Feelings of Worthlessness or Guilt
- Difficulty Concentrating
- Irritability, restlessness
- Physical Symptoms such as body aches, cramps etc.
- Thoughts of Death or Suicide or self-harm
- Withdrawal from Social Activities
- Feelings of Helplessness

It's important to remember that depression is a highly individualized experience, and not everyone with depression will exhibit the same symptoms. Moreover, the severity and duration of these symptoms can vary from person to person. If you or someone you know is experiencing these symptoms, seeking professional help and support is vital for managing and recovering from depression.

1.3.3 Is Depression the same in everyone?

As I said, depression is never a one-size-fits-all condition; it's more like an artist's palette with a myriad of colours and shades. The way depression manifests can be as unique as the individuals it affects in various aspects such as the below

Severity: Depression can range from mild to severe. In some cases, it may be a persistent feeling of sadness that lingers in the background, while in others, it can be an overwhelming and all-encompassing darkness.

Duration: For some, depression may be episodic, coming and going, while for others, it can be a chronic presence that persists for years.

Physical Symptoms: It's not just an emotional burden; depression can also bring physical symptoms like changes in appetite, sleep disturbances, and unexplained aches and pains.

Cognitive Symptoms: Depression can impact thinking, leading to self-critical thoughts, difficulty making decisions, and impaired concentration.

Motivational Changes: Some individuals with depression experience a loss of motivation, while others may have a strong desire to do things but find themselves unable to follow through.

Suicidal Thoughts: While not everyone with depression experiences these thoughts, some may have recurring thoughts of death or suicide or the self-harm

Psychotic Symptoms: In cases of severe depression, individuals may experience hallucinations or delusions, although this is less common.

Atypical Features: Atypical depression can include symptoms such as improved mood in response to positive events, excessive sleep, increased appetite, and a heavy sensation in the limbs.

Seasonal Patterns: Seasonal affective disorder (SAD) presents with recurrent depressive episodes during specific seasons, most commonly in the fall and winter. Have you ever heard of monsoon blues? Foggy weather bringing up a dull mood?

The variability of depression's expression underlines the importance of personalized and comprehensive treatment approaches. Understanding how depression uniquely affects an individual is essential for tailoring interventions to address their specific challenges and needs.

1.4 Stigma and Depression

Stigma refers to the negative attitudes, beliefs, and stereotypes that society holds towards certain individuals or groups based on characteristics, attributes, or conditions that they consider different, deviant, or socially undesirable. Stigma can lead to social exclusion, discrimination, and unfair treatment of these individuals or groups and, unfortunately depression is one of those conditions often surrounded by the stigma.

Stigma often arises from lack of knowledge, misconceptions, or fear of the unknown. It can be associated with a wide range of attributes, such as age, gender race, sexual orientation, marital status, pregnancy and maternity, religion or belief, disability, all of which are grouped as protected characteristics by the Equality Act UK 2010.

Stigmatized individuals often face prejudice, stereotypes, and discrimination, which can have profound and negative effects on their well-being, access to opportunities, and quality of life.

Stigma can manifest in various ways, including:

Social Isolation: People with depression may face social exclusion and isolation because of the misconception that they are "different" or that their condition is somehow contagious or undesirable. Have you noticed any of your family members/friends/relatives regularly avoiding to attend the functions/social gatherings/ meetings/ parties recently? Time to check if they're okay!

Negative Stereotypes: Stereotypes about individuals with depression can be damaging. They may be unfairly seen as weak, lazy, or as lacking willpower, but, in reality, depression is a complex condition that has nothing to do with these qualities.

Discrimination: In some cases, people with depression may face discrimination in areas such as employment, housing, or access to healthcare. Employers or landlords may discriminate against them based on the misconception that individuals with depression are unreliable or incapable.

Lack of Understanding: A lack of understanding about depression can lead to insensitive or dismissive comments such as "hey everything is going to be okay", "leave it, don't overthink", "time shall pass on". Ever heard of such or passed such comments?

This lack of empathy can deter individuals from seeking help or confiding in others.

Self-Stigma: People with depression sometimes internalize these societal attitudes, leading to self-stigmatization. They may feel ashamed or blame themselves for their condition, which can hinder their recovery and treatment-seeking.

The stigma surrounding depression can be a significant barrier to those who need help. It often discourages individuals from seeking treatment, sharing their experiences, or even acknowledging their condition to themselves. Reducing the stigma associated with depression is a crucial step in ensuring that individuals receive the support, understanding, and treatment they need to manage and recover from this mental health challenge.

Stigma surrounding mental health conditions like depression doesn't operate in isolation; it ripples through families, affecting not only the individual with depression but also their loved ones. Here's a closer look at the ripple effect of stigma within families:

Impact on Communication: Stigma can create a barrier to open and honest communication within families. Family members may avoid discussing the depressed individual's condition, which can hinder understanding and support.

Feelings of Guilt and Helplessness: Family members may experience guilt or helplessness when a loved one is dealing with depression. They might question if they did something to cause it or feel unable to alleviate their loved one's suffering.

Strained Relationships: Stigma can strain relationships within families. Misunderstandings, unspoken emotions, and frustration can build up, leading to a strain on family dynamics.

Isolation: Family members may feel isolated or alone in their efforts to support a loved one with depression, as they fear the judgment or lack of understanding from others outside the family.

Lack of Empathy: Stigma can affect family members' ability to empathize with the person with depression. They may struggle to comprehend the emotional pain and the impact it has on their loved one.

Blame and Misconceptions: Family members may inadvertently blame the individual with depression for their condition or hold misconceptions about the nature of mental health. This can lead to frustration and miscommunication.

Delayed Intervention: Stigma may lead to a delay in seeking help for the person with depression. Family members, influenced by societal stigmas, may discourage or avoid professional treatment, thinking they can handle it themselves.

The Cycle of Silence: The family's hesitation to discuss depression can perpetuate a cycle of silence and misunderstanding, which makes it difficult to break down stigma and foster a supportive environment.

1.5 Myths and facts around Depression

Depression is a widely misunderstood condition, and many myths and misconceptions surround it. Here are some common misconceptions about depression along with the facts that challenge them: Check if you too have any of those false beliefs!

Myth: Depression is just feeling sad, and it will pass.

Fact: Depression is a mental health disorder characterized by persistent feelings of sadness, hopelessness, and a range of other symptoms. It is not a fleeting emotion and often requires professional treatment.

Myth: Depression is a sign of personal weakness.

Fact: Depression is not a sign of weakness or a lack of willpower. It's a medical condition influenced by various factors, including genetics, brain chemistry, and life circumstances.

Myth: People with depression can "snap out of it" or should just "think positively."

Fact: Depression is not a choice, and positive thinking alone cannot cure it. It often requires professional treatment, which may include therapy and medication.

Myth: Only traumatic events can cause depression.

Fact: While life events can trigger depression, it can also be influenced by genetics, brain chemistry, and other factors. It's not exclusively linked to negative experiences.

Myth: Medication is the only treatment for depression.

Fact: Treatment for depression is multifaceted and can include therapy, lifestyle changes, support networks, and medication, depending on the individual's needs.

Myth: People with depression are always sad and can't have moments of happiness.

Fact: People with depression can experience moments of happiness, but these moments are often overshadowed by the persistent sadness and other symptoms of depression.

Myth: Depression is rare, and only a small number of people experience it.

Fact: Depression is one of the most common mental health disorders, affecting millions of people worldwide from all walks of life.

Myth: If someone is functioning well in their daily life, they can't have depression.

Fact: Many individuals with depression continue to function well in their daily lives, but they may be struggling internally. High-functioning depression is a real phenomenon.

Myth: Depression is a lifelong, untreatable condition.

Fact: Depression is treatable, and many individuals experience significant improvements with appropriate treatment, support, and lifestyle changes.

Myth: Depression doesn't affect children/teenagers

Fact: Depression can affect anyone regardless of age and unfortunately children/teenagers don't express

Myth: Educated and well settled individuals don't/shouldn't suffer depression

Fact: Properties, and educational qualifications, can't keep the mental conditions away

1.6 How to challenge misconceptions?

- **Educate Yourself:** Take the time to learn about depression, its causes, symptoms, and treatments. Understanding the condition is the first step in challenging stereotypes.

- **Promote Open Conversations:** Encourage open and non-judgmental conversations about mental health, including depression. Provide a safe space for individuals to share their experiences and feelings.

- **Share Personal Stories:** Sharing personal stories of lived experiences with depression can humanize the condition and challenge stereotypes. Hearing from individuals who have overcome depression can be inspiring.

- **Avoid Language that Reinforces Stigma:** Be mindful of the language you use. Avoid derogatory or stigmatizing terms when discussing depression. Use person-first language that emphasizes the individual, not the condition.

- **Emphasize that Depression is a Medical Condition:** Help others understand that depression is not a choice or a sign of personal weakness. It is a medical condition that can affect anyone.

- **Highlight Diverse Experiences:** Recognize that depression affects people differently. Highlight the diversity of experiences, including those who may not fit the stereotypical image of someone with depression.

- **Challenge Gender Stereotypes:** Combat gender-based stereotypes by acknowledging that depression can affect people of all genders, and it may manifest differently in different individuals.

- **Acknowledge the Intersection of Identities:** Understand that individuals with depression may have intersecting identities (e.g., race, sexuality, gender) that influence their experiences. Challenge stereotypes that intersect with these identities.

- **Promote Empathy:** Encourage empathy and active listening when discussing depression. Help others understand the emotional and psychological pain that individuals with depression may experience.

- **Support Mental Health Advocacy:** Get involved in mental health advocacy and support organizations that work to challenge stereotypes and reduce stigma. Participate in campaigns and events that promote mental health awareness.

- **Normalize Help-Seeking:** Normalize the act of seeking help for mental health issues, including depression. Encourage individuals to reach out to mental health professionals without fear of judgment.

- **Lead by Example:** Be a role model in challenging stereotypes. Your own attitudes and behaviours can influence those around you. Show empathy and understanding in your interactions with individuals who have depression.

Challenging stereotypes about depression is an ongoing effort that requires education, empathy, and open dialogue. By actively working to break down these stereotypes, you contribute to a more compassionate and supportive society for those dealing with depression.

I hope by now, it is clear that the depression isn't just a feeling of sadness but a complex medical condition that requires prompt treatment. The stereotypical society with negative attitudes makes it even more complex and I hope the commonest myths around the depression have been demystified. Step into the second section of this book for a detailed understanding of how depression manifests to create a more compassionate and supportive world for individuals living with depression.

A minute to reflect!

Think about the myths and misconceptions you've come across regarding depression. Are there any types that resonate with your experiences or those of someone you know? How these myths contributed to your misunderstanding and stigma?

2. THE DEPTH OF DEPRESSION

"Being around people isn't a sign of being unlonley"
-Dr. Sloka

In the process of understanding depression, let's now shift our focus on to recognizing the signs and symptoms, also learning about the causes and triggering factors. All since, **recognition is the key** to seeking/offering help and support.

Although a list of common signs and symptoms have been discussed in the section 1 for basic understanding, let's go a bit deeper understand how it presents in individuals.

2.1 RECOGNIZING THE SIGNS AND SYMPTOMS OF DEPRESSION

Several emotional, behavioural, and physical changes can be observed in individuals suffering from depression as below

2.1.1 Common Emotional Symptoms

Persistent Sadness: Individuals with depression often experience a deep and prolonged sense of sadness. This sadness isn't always related to a specific event and can last for weeks or months.

Irritability: Feelings of irritability, restlessness, or agitation can be prominent in depression, especially in men and younger individuals.

Difficulty Concentrating: Depression often impacts cognitive abilities, making it challenging to concentrate, make decisions, and remember things.

Feelings of Guilt or Worthlessness: People with depression may experience excessive guilt or feelings of worthlessness, often without a clear reason.

Thoughts of Death or Suicide: While not everyone with depression experiences this, thoughts of death or suicide can be a severe sign that requires immediate attention.

Pessimism: A negative outlook on the future, hopelessness, and a belief that things will never get better are often associated with depression.

Unexplained Crying: Frequent and unexplained bouts of crying can be a symptom of depression.

2.1.2 Behavioral Signs of Depression

Depression can manifest through various changes in behaviour. If you notice these behavioural signs in yourself or someone else, it might be an indicator of depression:

Social Withdrawal: Depression can make individuals withdraw from social interactions. They may avoid friends, family, and social gatherings, feeling like they can't muster the energy or interest to engage. This isolation can lead to a sense of loneliness and further exacerbate feelings of depression.

Reduced Activity: One of the hallmark signs of depression is a marked reduction in physical activity. People with depression may feel physically and mentally drained, as if even small tasks require immense effort. This lack of energy can make it difficult to complete daily responsibilities.

Neglected Responsibilities: Meeting responsibilities at work, school, or home can become increasingly challenging for individuals with depression. They may struggle to concentrate, meet deadlines, or complete tasks they once managed easily, leading to a sense of failure and eventually their self-worth is affected

Changes in Sleep Patterns: Sleep disturbances are common in depression. Some individuals may have trouble falling asleep or staying asleep (insomnia), while others might sleep excessively (hypersomnia). These sleep disruptions can further affect mood and energy levels.

Appetite Changes: Depression often affects eating habits. Some people may lose their appetite and have trouble eating, leading to weight loss. Others might turn to food for comfort, overeating and potentially gaining weight.

Substance Abuse: In an attempt to self-medicate or numb emotional pain, feel calmer, individuals with depression turn to alcohol or drugs that eventually becomes a habit and then addiction. Substance abuse can provide a temporary escape but exacerbates mental health issues in the long run.

Increased Irritability: Depression doesn't always manifest as sadness. Some individuals become easily irritated, short-tempered, or even angry in response to minor frustrations. This emotional volatility can strain relationships.

Self-Harm: In severe cases of depression, individuals may resort to self-destructive behaviours like self-harm. This harmful coping mechanism provides momentary relief from emotional pain but is dangerous and not a solution.

Neglect of Personal Hygiene: Individuals with depression may neglect personal care and hygiene routines, such as bathing, grooming, and dressing. This can be a visible outward sign of the inner struggles they're facing. Not a sign of laziness!

Reckless Behaviour: Some individuals with depression may engage in risky or impulsive activities without considering the consequences. This can include dangerous driving, substance abuse, or other actions that put their well-being at risk.

Avoidance of Enjoyable Activities: Anhedonia, or the inability to experience pleasure, is common in depression. People may lose interest in activities that previously brought them joy, making it difficult to find fulfilment in life. Check with them if they're okay!

These behavioural signs often interconnect with the emotional and cognitive symptoms of depression. Recognizing these changes in behaviour is a crucial first step in seeking help and support to manage and recover from depression.

Recall anyone with such symptoms in the past? Have you ever thought "oh they're eating more/less, sleeping more/don't sleep at all", they're always moody/lazy"? Hopefully you changed your perspective now.

2.1.3 Physical Symptoms to Watch For

Physical symptoms can also manifest alongside emotional and behavioural signs of depression. These can be indicators that someone is experiencing depressive symptoms:

Headaches: Individuals with depression often complain of frequent or persistent headaches, which can be tension-related.

Digestive Problems: Depression can affect the digestive system, leading to issues like stomach-aches, indigestion, or changes in bowel habits.

Body Aches: Unexplained body aches and pains, such as muscle soreness or joint discomfort, can accompany depression.

Fatigue: People with depression commonly report a profound sense of fatigue. It's not just being tired but a deep, all-encompassing weariness that persists, even after a full night's sleep.

Changes in Appetite and Weight: Depression can lead to alterations in eating habits. Some individuals may experience an increase in appetite and overeat, potentially leading to weight gain. Others might lose interest in food, resulting in weight loss.

Slowed Movement and Speech: In some cases, depression can lead to physical slowing, both in movements and speech. Individuals may appear physically and verbally lethargic, as if they are physically weighed down by their emotional state.

Sexual Dysfunction: Changes in libido, difficulties with sexual performance, and a decreased sense of satisfaction in intimate relationships.

If you or someone you know is experiencing these physical symptoms along with other signs of depression, please help them in seeking professional support. Depression is a treatable condition, and early intervention can lead to positive outcomes.

2.2 Red Flags to Look for- warning signs for suicide

Suicidal thoughts aren't just about "I want to die" but individuals can express it in different ways, as below and recognizing them as alarming signs is the most important step in preventing the loss of a loved one suffering from depression.

"I want to escape and disappear"

"I wish I could go to sleep and don't wake up"

"I am a burden to my parents/family"

"I wake up only for my kids"

"Who should I live for"?

"What's the purpose of my life"?

"Nobody needs me"

"Everyone would be better off without me"

The above statements aren't mere thoughts out of a general frustration but could be potential signs of them suffering in silence. High time to pay attention! Talking about suicide is another subject of taboo and lot of stigma runs around it to a level that even speaking out the word 'suicide' openly from mouth is also felt disturbing, or embarrassing for many. When you notice any such warning signs in people around, please speak to them openly about suicide. You could save a life!

2.3 Sadness and Depression- are they both same?

As explained in the earlier sections that the depression is a disorder having persistent feelings of sadness, often people mistake depression for sadness but it is not. It's important to understand the differences between them.

Sadness and clinical depression are two distinct emotional states

Sadness is a common and natural human emotion, clinical depression is a mental health condition.

Sadness is a temporary emotional state in reaction to certain stressors such as loss, disappointment, betrayal, while depression includes persistent sadness for extended periods of time.

Sadness is a subjective experience but depression needs a definitive diagnosis

Sadness involves transient mood changes but depression affects multiple areas such as social, personal, interpersonal, cognitive, behavioural, physical, mental and emotional domains.

Sadness is common in everyone's life for several reasons but it becomes a concern when it manifests as above explained signs and symptoms of depression.

2.4 What causes Depression?

It's often hard to point at a single reason as a cause because the potential causes of depression are multifactorial and may include biological, environmental, and psychosocial factors.

2.4.1 Biological Factors: Genetic Predisposition

Genetics, hormones, neurotransmitters, play an important role in the onset of depression.

Inherited Traits: Depression can run in families, suggesting a genetic component. If close family members, such as parents or siblings, have a history of depression, there may be a genetic predisposition.

Complex Inheritance: The genetic basis of depression is complex. It's not linked to a single gene but involves multiple genes that interact with each other and with environmental factors. This complexity makes it challenging to pinpoint specific genetic causes.

Susceptibility to Stress: Genetic factors may influence how an individual responds to stress. Some people with a genetic predisposition may be more susceptible to the negative effects of stress, which can trigger or exacerbate depression.

Neurotransmitter Function: Genetic variations can affect the functioning of neurotransmitters (chemical messengers in the brain), such as serotonin and dopamine. Changes in these neurotransmitters are linked to mood regulation and can contribute to depression.

Neurochemical imbalances are significant factors that can contribute to the development of depression. These factors are closely related and impact the functioning of the brain. Neurotransmitters are chemicals in the brain that facilitate communication between nerve cells. Common neurotransmitters associated with depression include serotonin, norepinephrine, and dopamine. An imbalance in these neurotransmitters can affect mood regulation, potentially leading to depression.

- **Serotonin Deficiency:** Low levels of serotonin are often linked to depressive symptoms. Serotonin is involved in regulating mood, sleep, and appetite. A deficiency can disrupt these processes, contributing to feelings of sadness and other depressive symptoms.

- **Norepinephrine Irregularities:** Norepinephrine is involved in the body's stress response. Abnormal norepinephrine levels may lead to a heightened stress response, which can increase the risk of depression.

- **Dopamine Dysfunction:** Dopamine is associated with pleasure and reward. Alterations in dopamine levels can impact the brain's reward system and may be linked to anhedonia, the inability to experience pleasure, which is a common symptom of depression.

2.4.2 Environmental Factors: Early Life Experiences

Early life experiences can significantly influence an individual's risk of developing depression. These experiences shape one's emotional and psychological well-being and can have long-lasting effects. Here's an explanation of how early life experiences can be potential causes of depression:

Adverse Childhood Events: Traumatic or adverse events during childhood, such as physical or emotional abuse, neglect, the loss of a parent, or exposure to domestic violence, can have a profound impact. These experiences may create emotional wounds that persist into adulthood and increase the risk of depression.

Attachment and Bonding: Early relationships with primary caregivers play a critical role in emotional development. A secure attachment to caregivers can provide a strong foundation for emotional well-being, while disrupted or insecure attachments may contribute to emotional difficulties and vulnerability to depression.

Childhood Bullying: Experiences of bullying or peer victimization during childhood can lead to feelings of social isolation, low self-esteem, and psychological distress, all of which are risk factors for depression.

Chronic Stress: Growing up in an environment marked by chronic stress, such as poverty, neighbourhood violence, or parental substance abuse, can lead to ongoing stress reactions and a higher likelihood of depression.

Parental Mental Health: Children raised by parents with mental health issues, especially untreated or poorly managed conditions, are at an increased risk of developing their own mental health problems, including depression.

Loss and Grief: The loss of a loved one, especially during childhood or adolescence, can be emotionally challenging and may trigger the onset of depressive symptoms.

Parental Modelling: Children often learn emotional coping strategies and behaviours from their parents. If parents have maladaptive ways of dealing with stress or emotional difficulties, their children may adopt similar patterns, potentially leading to depression.

Negative Self-Image: Childhood experiences that consistently reinforce a negative self-image or feelings of inadequacy can contribute to low self-esteem and a heightened risk of depression.

Social Isolation: If a child experiences social isolation, exclusion, or difficulties forming peer relationships, it can lead to feelings of loneliness and increase the risk of depression.

2.4.3 Psychosocial factors

Psychosocial factors include negative self-image, low self-esteem, rumination, low emotional clarity.

2.5 The Common Triggers

2.5.1 The Role of Life Transitions

Life transitions, both major and minor, can serve as triggers for depressive episodes. These transitions mark significant changes in one's life circumstances, and the adjustment process can be emotionally challenging. Here's an explanation of the role of life transitions in triggering depressive episodes:

Adjustment Stress: Life transitions often bring about stress as individuals adapt to new situations or roles. Whether it's starting a new job, moving to a new city, or experiencing a change in relationship status, the stress of adjustment can trigger or exacerbate depressive symptoms.

Loss and Grief: Some life transitions involve loss, such as the death of a loved one, the end of a significant relationship, or the loss of a job. Grief and mourning can lead to depressive symptoms, especially when the loss is profound.

Identity and Self-Esteem: Life transitions can challenge one's sense of identity and self-esteem. For example, retirement or working in a profession that is not aligned with passion may lead to a loss of identity tied to one's career, and adjusting to a new role as a parent can be emotionally overwhelming. These changes in self-perception can contribute to depressive episodes.

Uncertainty: Life transitions often introduce uncertainty about the future. This uncertainty can create anxiety and distress, which, when prolonged or severe, may lead to depressive symptoms.

Social Isolation: Some life transitions, like relocation or retirement, can result in social isolation. The loss of social connections can lead to feelings of loneliness and sadness, increasing the risk of depression.

Financial Changes: Financial stress can be a significant outcome of certain life transitions, such as job loss or divorce. Economic difficulties can be emotionally distressing and contribute to depressive episodes.

Health-Related Transitions: A diagnosis of a chronic illness or a significant health event can be a life-altering transition. Coping with health-related changes can trigger feelings of sadness and uncertainty.

2.5.2 Relationship Struggles and Loss

Relationship struggles and loss, whether in personal or interpersonal contexts, can serve as powerful triggers for depressive episodes.

Conflict and Stress: Ongoing conflicts within relationships, such as with a partner, family member, or friend, can lead to chronic stress. This stress, when left unaddressed, can contribute to depressive symptoms.

Communication Difficulties: Poor communication, misunderstandings, or a lack of emotional connection in relationships can result in feelings of frustration and isolation, which are risk factors for depression.

Loss of a Loved One: The death or loss of a close friend or family member can trigger intense grief and sadness. If the grieving process is prolonged or complicated, it may lead to depressive symptoms.

Divorce or Breakup: The end of a significant romantic relationship, such as divorce or a breakup, can be emotionally distressing. The loss of a partner, along with the associated changes in one's life circumstances, can lead to depressive episodes.

Low Self-Esteem: Negative experiences within relationships can erode self-esteem and self-worth. Individuals who perceive themselves as unworthy or unlovable due to relationship difficulties are at greater risk of developing depression.

Stressful Family Dynamics: Struggles within family dynamics, including issues related to parental relationships or conflicts with children, can create a chronic and emotionally taxing environment that increases the risk of depression.

Infidelity and Betrayal: Experiencing betrayal, such as infidelity in a romantic relationship or betrayal by a trusted friend, can result in deep emotional wounds and contribute to depression.

Lack of Support: A lack of emotional support or empathy from relationships during challenging times can exacerbate depressive symptoms. Feeling unheard or invalidated can intensify emotional distress.

It's important to recognize that relationship struggles and loss are common life experiences, and they can be emotionally distressing for anyone. Seeking support from friends, family, or a mental health professional can be instrumental in navigating these challenges and addressing depressive symptoms. Early intervention and effective coping strategies are key to managing and preventing depression related to relationship difficulties and loss.

2.5.3 Substance Abuse and Its Connection to Depression

Substance abuse can play a complex role in triggering depressive episodes. The relationship between substance use and depression is often bidirectional, with each issue influencing and exacerbating the other. Individuals often depend on pleasure obtained from substance use but the reward is only temporary and leads to several mental health challenges like addiction, depressive symptoms.

Chemical Imbalances: Substance abuse, particularly of smoking, cannabis or alcohol, can disrupt the balance of neurotransmitters in the brain. This chemical imbalance can affect mood regulation and lead to symptoms of depression.

Withdrawal Symptoms: When individuals who regularly use substances try to quit or reduce their use, they may experience withdrawal symptoms. These symptoms can include mood swings, anxiety, and deep sadness, resembling depressive symptoms.

Interference with Treatment: Substance abuse can hinder the effectiveness of depression treatment. It can make it challenging for individuals to engage in therapy or adhere to medication regimens.

2.5.4 Co-occurring Mental Health Disorders

Co-occurring mental health disorders, also known as comorbidities, can be significant triggers for depressive episodes in the following way:

Interaction of Symptoms: When an individual has multiple mental health disorders, the symptoms of one condition can interact with and exacerbate the symptoms of another. This interaction can intensify emotional distress, potentially leading to depressive episodes.

Shared Risk Factors: Many mental health disorders share common risk factors, such as genetic predisposition or early-life trauma. These shared risk factors can increase an individual's vulnerability to multiple conditions, including depression.

Self-Stigma and Shame: Co-occurring disorders may lead to self-stigma or feelings of shame, which can contribute to depressive symptoms. Individuals may blame themselves for their mental health challenges, leading to low self-esteem and sadness.

Complicated Treatment: Managing multiple mental health conditions can be complex. The need for multiple treatments and medications, as well as potential interactions between them, can create stress and lead to depressive symptoms.

Interference with Daily Functioning: Co-occurring disorders can interfere with daily functioning, affecting one's ability to work, maintain relationships, and enjoy life. This interference can contribute to depressive episodes.

Isolation and Social Withdrawal: Individuals with co-occurring disorders may withdraw from social interactions due to stigma or difficulties in managing their conditions. This isolation can increase feelings of loneliness and sadness, further triggering depressive symptoms.

Physical Health Consequences: Some mental health conditions can lead to physical health issues such as hypertension (high blood pressure), diabetes (high blood sugar), and dyslipidaemia (altered blood cholesterol levels). The physical consequences, along with the emotional distress related to these conditions, can contribute to depressive episodes.

A minute to reflect!

Reflect on the signs and symptoms of depression and think about potential warning signs or triggers that you may have overlooked in yourself or others. If you remembered someone, quickly check on them!

3. PATHWAYS TO HEALING

> *"A tumor of despair and thoughts can be treated with radiation of comfort,*
> *If a little support can be an invisible string of connection, friends and family can become all time therapists" - Dr. Sloka*

Depression is a mental illness, but it is also a highly treatable condition. Seeking professional help is often the pivotal first step towards healing. This section will provide insights into why professional guidance is essential, how to find the right mental health provider, and what to expect during the initial phases of seeking help, the vast landscape of treatment options, from therapy and medication to alternative and complementary approaches. Yet, the journey towards recovery is not without its challenges and so we'll explore strategies to overcome these obstacles, making the process of healing more accessible and manageable.

3.1 The Mental Health Specialists

Many of you lack familiarity with mental health professionals. You may only recognize terms like psychiatrist or psychologist and often struggle to differentiate between them or comprehend other mental health specialists. Let's explore the realm of mental health experts in more detail

- **Psychiatrist:**

Psychiatrists are medical doctors who can diagnose and treat mental health conditions, including depression. They can prescribe medication and provide a range of treatment options.

- **Psychologist:**

Psychologists hold advanced degrees in psychology/mental health (mind and the behaviour) and provide therapy and counselling for individuals with mental health concerns. They conduct assessments and offer various types of interventions in the form of psychotherapies depending on the condition.

- **Medical Social Worker:**

Medical social workers are trained in providing counselling services to individuals and families. They often specialize in addressing social and environmental factors that contribute to mental health issues.

- **Mental Health Counsellor:**

Mental health counsellors are trained to offer therapy and counselling to individuals and groups. They help individuals manage and overcome mental health challenges, including depression.

- **Marriage and Family Therapist:**

Marriage and family therapists specialize in addressing relationship and family-related mental health issues. They provide therapy to individuals, couples, and families to improve relationships and mental well-being.

- **Art Therapist:**

Art therapists use creative processes, such as art, to help individuals express and understand their emotions and mental health concerns. This form of therapy can be beneficial for those who may find it challenging to express themselves verbally.

- **Occupational Therapist:**

Occupational therapists help individuals develop the skills needed to engage in daily life activities and improve their mental health and well-being. They work with individuals to enhance their functional abilities.

- **Peer Support Specialist:**

Peer support specialists have personal experience with mental health challenges and recovery. They offer support, empathy, and guidance to individuals facing similar challenges, serving as role models for recovery.

- **Substance Abuse Counsellor:**

These counsellors specialize in helping individuals with substance use disorders, which can often co-occur with depression. They provide counselling and support for addiction and its impact on mental health.

Each type of mental health professional brings unique skills and approaches to the table, and the choice of the right professional often depends on an individual's specific needs, preferences, and the nature of their mental health concerns. The journey of healing often includes a collaborative care involving different mental health professionals.

3.2 The Role of Mental Health Team

Healthcare professionals play a vital role in the treatment of depression, providing essential support and guidance to individuals on their journey to recovery. Their roles and contributions include;

- **Assessment and Diagnosis:**

Healthcare professionals, such as psychiatrists, psychologists, and primary care physicians, conduct thorough assessments using standardized tools to diagnose depression. They evaluate the severity of symptoms, rule out other potential causes to make a concrete diagnosis

- **Treatment Planning:**

Based on the diagnosis, healthcare professionals develop personalized treatment plans. The plans may include therapy, medication, or a combination of both, tailored to the individual's unique needs and preferences.

- **Medication Management:**

Psychiatrists, some primary care physicians, and certified pharmacists are qualified to prescribe and manage antidepressant medications. They monitor the effectiveness of medications, adjust dosages as needed, and address any side effects or concerns.

- **Psychotherapy:**

Psychologists, therapists, and counsellors provide various forms of psychotherapy, such as cognitive-behavioural therapy (CBT) or interpersonal therapy. These therapies help individuals understand and manage their depressive symptoms, develop coping strategies, and make positive behavioural changes.

- **Support and Encouragement:**

Healthcare professionals offer emotional support and encouragement, fostering a safe and non-judgmental space for individuals to discuss their feelings, experiences, and progress. This support is essential in reducing the isolation that often accompanies depression.

- **Education and Information:**

Professionals educate individuals about depression, its causes, and the available treatment options. They help patients and their families understand the condition and the rationale behind the chosen treatment plan.

- **Monitoring Progress:**

Healthcare providers regularly assess the progress of treatment, ensuring that it aligns with the individual's goals and that adjustments are made as necessary. They track symptom improvements and any setbacks.

- **Crisis Intervention:**

In cases of severe depression or when individuals express thoughts of self-harm or suicide, healthcare professionals provide immediate crisis intervention and safety planning. They may coordinate hospitalization or intensive care when required.

- **Collaboration with Other Specialists:**

In complex cases, healthcare professionals collaborate with other specialists, such as social workers, addiction counsellors, or occupational therapists, to address the diverse needs of individuals with depression.

- **Medication Education:**

Professionals provide information about prescribed medications, dosing, potential side effects, drug to drug and drug to food interactions, how to manage the side effects, and the importance of adherence. They address concerns and ensure individuals have a clear understanding of their medication regimen.

- **Promoting Lifestyle Changes:**

Healthcare professionals often recommend lifestyle changes that can complement treatment, such as regular exercise, a balanced diet, and stress management techniques. These changes contribute to overall well-being.

- **Long-term Support:**

The role of healthcare professionals extends beyond the acute phase of treatment. They provide long-term support, helping individuals maintain their mental health, prevent relapse, and build resilience.

- **Advocacy and Awareness:**

Healthcare professionals contribute to the reduction of mental health stigma and advocate for policies and practices that support individuals with depression. They work to increase public awareness and understanding of mental health.

In short, seeking professional guidance is not just a smart choice; it can be a life-changing one and is so crucial for those dealing with depression. Their expertise, compassion, and dedication empower individuals to overcome the challenges of depression and regain their emotional well-being.

3.3 The Process of Diagnosis

The diagnostic process includes a series of assessments and evaluations conducted by mental health professionals to determine whether an individual is experiencing depression, the nature and severity of their symptoms, and to rule out other potential causes for their emotional distress. This process typically includes:

- **Clinical Interviews:**

Healthcare professionals, such as psychiatrists or psychologists, conduct in-depth interviews with the individual to gather information about their symptoms, medical history, and personal background. These interviews help in understanding the individual's experiences and emotional state.

- **Symptom Assessment:**

Professionals use standardized tools or questionnaires to assess the presence and severity of depressive symptoms. These assessments may include questions about mood, sleep patterns, appetite, energy levels, and thoughts of self-harm.

- **Diagnostic Criteria:**

The diagnostic process involves determining if the individual's symptoms align with the criteria outlined in diagnostic manuals such as the DSM-5 (Diagnostic and Statistical Manual of Mental Disorders). Specialists use certain standard scales to assess the criteria and to receive a diagnosis of depression, specific criteria related to the duration and intensity of symptoms must be met.

- **Medical Evaluation:**

It is essential to rule out potential medical conditions that can mimic or contribute to depressive symptoms. A physical examination and laboratory tests may be conducted to identify any underlying health issues.

- **Differential Diagnosis:**

Professionals consider alternative explanations for the symptoms, as there are various mental health conditions and emotional distress that may share similarities with depression. They aim to distinguish depression from other conditions like bipolar disorder, anxiety disorders, or grief.

- **Collateral Information:**

Gathering information from the individual's family or close contacts can provide valuable insights into the duration and impact of their symptoms.

- **Assessment of Functioning:**

Healthcare professionals evaluate how the symptoms of depression are affecting the individual's daily life, including their work, relationships, and overall well-being.

- **Cultural and Contextual Considerations:**

It's important to consider an individual's cultural background and life circumstances, as these factors can influence the experience of depression and the expression of symptoms.

- **Treatment Planning and monitoring progress:**

Based on the information collected during the diagnostic process, healthcare professionals develop a personalized treatment plan. This plan may include therapy, medication, or other interventions to address the individual's specific needs, follow up schedules to track and monitor the progress.

- **The Collaborative Approach: Involving Loved Ones**

When someone is going through a tough time with depression, it's not just their journey; it's a team effort that involves the people who care about them. You don't have to fix the things but just be there for them giving reassurance that they're not alone in the journey, show concerns, talk openly about their feelings, ask/involve in the treatment plans, different therapies, encouraging self-care, being patient, and celebrating the progress.

3.4 Treatment Modalities

Treatment modalities refer to the various approaches, methods, and techniques used in the medical or therapeutic treatment of a particular condition, illness, or health issue. These modalities can encompass a wide range of interventions and strategies aimed at addressing different aspects of the condition, managing symptoms, promoting healing, and improving overall well-being.

In the context of mental health and depression, treatment modalities may include **psychotherapy** (talk therapy), **drug therapy**, lifestyle modifications, and complementary therapies, all of which are employed to help individuals manage and alleviate their depressive symptoms. The choice of treatment modality or a combination of modalities is often based on the individual's specific needs, the severity of their condition, and their preferences, as well as the recommendations of healthcare professionals.

3.4.1 Psychotherapy (Talk Therapy)

Imagine sitting down and having a friendly conversation with someone who is trained to help you feel better! That's what psychotherapy, often called talk therapy, is all about. It helps not only feel better but understand the root causes. There are different types of psychotherapies such as interpersonal therapy, Cognitive Behavioural Therapy (CBT), mindfulness, Dialectical Behaviour Therapy (DBT), animal assisted therapy, arts therapy, and play therapy.

Psychotherapy sessions can be short term or long term and both the patient and therapist are actively involved, goals are discussed by both together.

Here's how it works:

- **Sharing Feelings and Thoughts:**

In therapy, you get the opportunity to express your innermost feelings and thoughts. It's like opening a door to your emotions, allowing them to flow freely. This safe and judgment-free space provides you with the freedom to discuss what's on your mind, no matter how big or small. It's a bit like taking off a heavy backpack of emotions and laying them out for examination.

- **Active Listening:**

The therapist isn't just any listener; they're a skilled, attentive, and compassionate one. They pay close attention to every word you say, as if your words are pieces of a puzzle they're putting together. They ask questions, not to interrogate, but to understand your perspective.

- **Exploring Challenges:**

Together with your therapist, it's like going on a tour to explore the challenges you're facing. Think of it as an adventure, where you navigate through the twists and turns of your emotions. You might uncover why you feel a certain way or unravel the threads of past experiences. It's a bit like archaeologists excavating the layers of your life to uncover hidden treasures of understanding.

- **Learning Coping Skills:**

Your therapist equips you with a set of tools and techniques to manage your emotions and deal with tough situations. It's like getting a toolkit for your mind and heart. These skills can include strategies for handling stress, strategies for changing negative thought patterns, and ways to build resilience.

- **Setting Goals:**

In therapy, you and your therapist work together to define what success looks like for you. These goals become your guiding stars, lighting your way as you navigate your journey to well-being.

- **Privacy and Confidentiality:**

Everything shared in therapy is locked in a vault of confidentiality. It's like having an impenetrable fortress for your secrets. You can speak your truth, your fears, and your hopes without worry. This secure space allows you to be completely honest and vulnerable, knowing your personal information remains protected.

3.4.2 Drug Therapy

Drug therapy, also known as pharmacological therapy, involves a qualified Psychiatrist or a practitioner prescribing medicines which includes antidepressants to treat the condition.

- **What Medication Does?**

Medications for depression work by increasing the levels of neurotransmitters such as serotonin, norepinephrine in your brain that play a significant role in mood regulation. By doing this, they aims to restore the balance of these mood regulating chemicals in the brain to alleviate depressive symptoms.

- **Types of Medications:**

There are different types of medications used to treat depression. The most common ones include:

- **Antidepressants:** These are the primary medications for depression. There are different classes of antidepressants such as selective serotonin reuptake inhibitors (SSRIs), serotonin-norepinephrine reuptake inhibitors (SNRIs), Mono Amine Oxidase Inhibitors (MAOI) and others. They work by increasing the availability of certain neurotransmitters in the brain each class of drugs working differently

- **Mood Stabilizers**: Sometimes, mood stabilizers like lithium are used for specific types of depression.

- **Antipsychotic Medications:** In some cases, especially when depression has psychotic features, antipsychotic medications may be prescribed in combination with other antidepressants. Few of the commonly used antipsychotics are Quetiapine, Risperidone, Olanzapine, haloperidol, chlorpromazine.

- **Prescribing and Monitoring:**

Medications for depression are prescribed by a qualified healthcare professional, typically a psychiatrist. The choice of medication depends on various factors, including the type and severity of depression, the individual's medical history, and any potential side effects. Your doctor may ask for certain parameters such as blood counts, blood glucose, thyroid function, kidney and liver function, and blood cholesterol levels to be tested before prescribing some medications and also during follow up because of their potential to affect other body systems. Therefore it's crucial to follow the prescribed regimen, get necessary investigations done as advised and attend regular follow-up appointments to monitor progress and make any necessary adjustments in the doses, frequency or duration of the treatment.

- **Time to Effect:**

Medicines are not magical elements to heal depression instantly and if that is your expectation, I am sorry as this is not what you wanted to know probably, but the reality is that antidepressants often take a few weeks to start showing their full effect. During this time, some individuals may not experience immediate relief from their symptoms, but it's essential to continue taking the medication as directed. Patience along with adherence to therapy is the key!

- **Combination Therapy:**

In some cases, a healthcare professional may recommend a combination of medication and psychotherapy for more comprehensive treatment. This approach can provide both immediate symptom relief and long-term coping strategies.

- **Side Effects:**

Like all medications, antidepressants can have side effects. These can vary from person to person and from one medication to another. Common side effects may include dizziness, drowsiness, dry mouth, or changes in appetite.

It's essential to discuss potential side effects with your doctor or a qualified drug therapist.

- **Stopping Medication:**

Do not stop any medication without the advice from your doctor. Abruptly discontinuing medication can lead to withdrawal symptoms or a return of depressive symptoms. Tapering off the medication is usually recommended to minimize these risks and the tapering plan is guided by your doctor. So, do not attempt to take your own decisions to stop the medications.

- **Duration of Treatment:**

The duration of medication treatment varies from person to person. Some individuals may only need medication for a specific period to manage a single episode of depression, while others may require long-term or even lifelong treatment.

- **Maintenance Therapy:**

For individuals with recurrent depression, maintenance therapy may be recommended to prevent future episodes. This may involve continuing to take a lower dose of the medication even when feeling well.

- **Individualized Care: sharing is caring doesn't apply to drugs**

It is often observed that patients share their medications when they notice similar symptoms in their family members or friends for various reasons such as intent to help, similar symptoms mean the same diagnosis and so the same medication, or to bypass visiting the doctor.

Sometimes, it is also seen that patients follow advices from their friends or relatives to stop or change the medicine or alter the dosing pattern because their doctor has done those changes for them

Medication treatment is highly individualized. What works best for one person may not be suitable for another. So, do not share the medication and do not make changes in your treatment on your own. It's essential to work closely with your healthcare provider to find the right medication and dosage that suits your needs.

Medication is a valuable tool in the comprehensive treatment of depression. When used in conjunction with other therapies, such as psychotherapy, it can be a crucial element in helping individuals regain their emotional well-being and improve their quality of life. Always consult with a qualified healthcare provider to discuss your specific needs and treatment options.

3.4.3 Lifestyle Changes and Behavioral Interventions (Instant mood up lifters)

The interventions explained below often serve as natural antidepressants or instant mood up lifters. The power of these lifestyle changes is often under estimated. Practice them consistently and you'll observe that these changes contribute towards a holistic approach to managing depression and promote your mental health and well-being. These are naturally therapeutic.

- **Good food equals to Good Mood:**

The phrase "Good food equals to Good Mood" isn't just a social media tagline but, food certainly helps to keep mood levels on the top. A well-balanced diet rich in nutrients can positively impact mood and energy levels. Certain foods, such as those containing omega-3 fatty acids, can have a beneficial effect on brain health. Also other nutrients such as Iron, Vitamin B12, folic acid either in the form of supplements or through the diet help maintain the optimum serotonin levels.

- **Movement for Mood:**

Physical activity is one of the best natural mood lifters. If you ever want to instantly elevate your mood, move! Shake your body, move your hips and hands, tap your feet and rotate your shoulders and knees. Body movement in the form of regular exercise releases endorphins, which are often called "feel-good" hormones. Regular work out isn't just for physical body but keeps you mentally fit and healthy. Benefits of physical activity on mental health is beyond the scope of this little paragraph but you don't need to end up paying for expensive gym memberships; engaging in any form of physical activity such as even a short walk in the garden, spot jogging, mountain climbing, stretching, swimming, can help reduce symptoms of depression and improve overall mental health.

- **Sleep Hygiene:**

Establishing healthy sleep patterns is crucial for managing depression. Sleep disruptions can exacerbate depressive symptoms. Implementing good sleep hygiene practices, such as maintaining a consistent sleep schedule and creating a restful sleep environment, can be highly beneficial.

- **Stress Reduction:**

Chronic stress can contribute to the development and exacerbation of depression. Learning stress-reduction techniques like mindfulness (bringing attention to present moment), meditation, relaxation exercises, making some arts and crafts, can help individuals manage stress and maintain emotional well-being.

- **Social Connections: but not addiction to social media!**

Isolation can worsen depressive symptoms. Building and maintaining social connections, even in small ways, is essential. This doesn't mean to say you spend your time on social media but rather to engage with friends, family, or even support groups within the community which can provide emotional support and a sense of belonging.

- **Structured Routine:**

Establishing a daily routine can provide a sense of stability and predictability. It helps individuals stay on track with daily tasks, add discipline to a day, and maintain a sense of purpose.

- **Setting Realistic Goals:**

Creating achievable goals, both short-term and long-term, can provide a sense of purpose and accomplishment. Your goals for a day can be as small as making your bed as you wake up in the morning, doing dishes without leaving for next day, eating meals on time, sleeping on time, not avoiding a shower, tidying up your room and wardrobe, not missing the appointments, bringing groceries or even making a set number of steps for a day. Success in accomplishing these small and set goals for a day can boost self-esteem and motivation to create further goals.

- **Avoiding Substance Abuse:**

Substance abuse, including excessive alcohol or drug use, I know, can bring up a bit of a pleasure and numb the emotional distress but remember, it is only for a short term relief. In reality, they worsen depressive symptoms and so say a big no to alcohol, tobacco smoking, e-cigarettes, or any other drugs that are giving you an instant pleasure.

Avoiding or addressing substance abuse is crucial for mental well-being.

- **Ongoing Self-Care:**

Managing depression is not a one-time effort but an ongoing journey. Give yourself a treat of getting a body massage, nails and hair done, a good skin care. Consistently practicing healthy lifestyle habits and behavioural interventions is key to maintaining emotional well-being.

- **Hobbies:**

Hobbies such as reading a novel of your interesting genre, watching a comedy show, listening to your favourite music, writing letters or drawing help instantly elevate your mood levels. Try them!

The holistic approach to depression recognizes the multifaceted nature of this condition and offers a well-rounded strategy for understanding, managing, and ultimately overcoming it. By considering the physical, emotional, social, and lifestyle aspects of depression, it provides a complete and more effective path to recovery and long-term mental well-being.

3.5 But! What stops us?

Seeking professional help and navigating treatment options for depression can be challenging due to various barriers. Recognizing these barriers is crucial to address them effectively. Here are some potential challenges and barriers individuals may face when seeking help for depression:

3.5.1 Stigma as a Barrier to Seeking Help

Stigma is a significant and pervasive barrier that prevents many individuals from seeking help for depression and other mental health conditions. Stigma can take various forms, and its effects are far-reaching. Do you know how stigma acts as a barrier to seeking help?

The "Macho" Myth: In some cultures, and societal groups, there exists a harmful notion that equates mental health struggles, including depression, with weakness.

Have you ever encountered remarks like, "Hey, why are you crying like a girl?" or "Come on, be strong, you're not a girl!" These statements not only associate depression with weakness but also discourage men from expressing their emotions openly, fostering a notion of masculinity that inhibits vulnerability. Furthermore, such comments indirectly reinforce stereotypes suggesting that women are inherently weak and expected to display emotions such as sadness and tears. This gender-specific stigma can prevent men from reaching out for support, exacerbating their depression in silence.

The Workplace Dilemma: The workplace can be a breeding ground for stigma. Individuals may fear disclosing their mental health condition to their employers or colleagues due to concerns about job security, discrimination, or perceived incompetence. This workplace stigma can hinder individuals from accessing the necessary support.

Cultural and Religious Stigma: Cultural beliefs and religious teachings can influence how individuals perceive mental health issues. Some cultures may stigmatize mental health conditions, associating them with shame or disgrace. In certain religious communities, individuals may feel that their faith should be sufficient to alleviate their mental suffering, leading to hesitance in seeking professional help.

The Mask of Perfectionism: Perfectionism can exacerbate stigma. Some individuals, driven by a need to appear flawless, may fear that seeking help for depression will shatter their image of perfection. This self-imposed expectation can lead to denial and hinder access to mental health support. Understand that there is nothing wrong in being imperfect in some areas of life, you can learn from imperfections and grow up, and you don't need to carry a burden of perfection.

Fear of Psychiatric Hospitals: This is often the biggest stigma we see all around. The psychiatric hospitals are often treated as places of imprisonment or punishment and this is causing fear, guilty and stigma. Individuals may avoid seeking help for depression out of concerns about being hospitalized involuntarily.

Celebrities and Misrepresentation: The public image of celebrities who struggle with mental health issues can sometimes reinforce stigma. Media misrepresentations or sensationalized stories may contribute to misconceptions about mental health treatment, making it difficult for individuals to seek help without fearing public judgment.

Perception of "Normal": Some individuals may mistakenly believe that feeling depressed is a "normal" part of life or that they can overcome it on their own. This perception can lead to self-doubt and delay in seeking professional help.

Perceived Burden on Others: Individuals with depression may worry that sharing their struggles with loved ones will burden them or strain relationships. This concern can lead to isolation and reluctance to seek help.

Generational Stigma: Stigma can be perpetuated across generations, with older family members passing down negative beliefs about mental health to younger generations. This generational stigma can hinder open discussions about depression and mental health support.

3.5.2 Financial and Access Barriers

Financial and access barriers present substantial challenges for individuals seeking help for depression. These barriers can limit the availability and affordability of mental health services, creating obstacles to accessing the support needed.

Limited Access to Services:

In many regions, there's a shortage of mental health providers, particularly in rural and underserved areas. This scarcity of mental health services can result in long wait times for appointments or difficulty finding a provider who is accepting new patients.

High Treatment Costs:

Mental health treatment, including therapy and medication, can become expensive. Without adequate insurance coverage, individuals may face substantial out-of-pocket expenses, making treatment unaffordable for many.

Lack of Insurance:

A significant barrier to accessing mental health services is the absence of health insurance. Without insurance coverage, individuals are often unable to access affordable mental health care, leaving them without essential support.

Geographical Barriers:

Geographic location can be a barrier to accessing mental health care. Individuals living in remote or rural areas may need to travel long distances to reach a mental health provider, adding additional costs and time constraints.

Language and Cultural Barriers:

Language and cultural differences can limit access to mental health services. Individuals who speak languages other than the predominant one in their region may struggle to find providers who can communicate effectively or understand their cultural background.

3.5.3 Medication Concerns and Side Effects

Medication concerns and potential side effects are valid and common challenges that individuals face when seeking help for depression. These concerns can create hesitance or reluctance to pursue medication as part of their treatment plan and adhere to the medication as prescribed.

Fear of Side Effects:

One of the primary concerns individuals have when considering medication for depression is the fear of side effects. They worry about how these side effects might affect their daily lives, well-being, or overall health.

Misconceptions about Medication:

Some individuals may hold misconceptions about psychiatric medications, such as believing they are addictive or that they will fundamentally change their personality. These misconceptions can lead to hesitation in trying medication.

Stigma and Medication:

Stigma surrounding psychiatric medication can deter individuals from considering it as a viable treatment option. They may worry about being perceived as "mentally ill" or "dependent" on medication, contributing to self-stigmatization.

Duration:

Finding the right medication and dosage can involve a period of trial and error. Individuals may be concerned about the time it takes to determine the most effective treatment, as well as potential side effects during this process. It's also a common misconception that psychiatric conditions need a long term therapy and people avoid taking medicines with this fear of long term treatment.

Perception of Medication as a "Last Resort":

Some individuals view medication as a last resort, only to be considered when other treatment options have failed. This perception can delay the initiation of medication, potentially prolonging suffering.

Balancing Medication with Other Treatments:

Many individuals receive a combination of treatments for depression, which may include therapy, lifestyle changes, and medication. Balancing these treatments and understanding their respective roles can be a concern.

Impact on Daily Life:

Some individuals may worry that the medication may affect their daily functioning, including cognitive abilities, energy levels, or emotional responsiveness. These concerns can lead to hesitation.

Medication Non-Adherence:

The fear of side effects or concerns about medication can lead to non-adherence, where individuals do not take their medication as prescribed, reducing its effectiveness.

Weight Gain and Body Image Concerns:

Certain antidepressants can cause weight gain, which can be distressing for individuals who have concerns about body image or have struggled with eating disorders.

Potential Withdrawal Effects: -

Discontinuing medication can lead to withdrawal effects for some individuals. The fear of experiencing withdrawal symptoms may dissuade them from considering medication.

3.6 Family, the First Support Group

Do you know that your family can be the first and the biggest support group in helping you overcome the depression? The involvement and support of family members can play a significant role in the treatment and recovery process for an individual with depression in various aspects of the journey.

3.6.1 Supporting Treatment Adherence

Ensuring treatment adherence is a critical aspect of managing depression, and the family plays an essential role in supporting their loved one's commitment to their treatment plan in multiple ways as below

1. Medication Management:

Family members can assist in medication management by helping their loved one establish a consistent routine for taking prescribed medications. This includes setting reminders, organizing pillboxes, and ensuring the medications are refilled as needed.

2. Understanding Medication:

Educating themselves about the prescribed medication can help family members understand its purpose, potential side effects, and the expected timeline for improvement. This knowledge can make them better prepared to address concerns or questions.

3. Encouragement and Positive Reinforcement:

Family members can provide ongoing encouragement and positive reinforcement. Recognizing the individual's efforts and progress can motivate them to continue with treatment.

4. Monitoring Side Effects:

Family members can keep an eye on the potential side effects, and report them to the healthcare providers. Family members can communicate any changes or concerns their loved one experiences, facilitating timely adjustments to the treatment plan.

5. Involvement in Therapy:

If the treatment plan includes therapy, family members can attend sessions or participate in family therapy. This involvement can enhance communication, understanding, and the effectiveness of therapy. More than all, it brings a "my family is there for me"- sense of belongingness to the individual.

6. Covert administration of medicines:

Most often patients are reluctant to take the medicines and the families try to administer in the disguised form by hiding them in the food or drink by crushing the medicines. This is called covert administration and is not to be a routinely practiced strategy. It involves medico-legal implications and to be administered only if the patient lacks the capacity to make their decisions about their health and medicines. Also, not all medicines are suitable for crushing since, when they are crushed they tend to either release the dose all at once and results in side effects or the medicines do not act in an intended way. So, check the suitability of medication before covertly administering with your doctor or a drug specialist and only under circumstances where it is deemed to be extremely important in the interests of patient safety, covert medication administration can be done following proper guidance from the healthcare professional.

3.6.2 Communicating with Healthcare Providers

Effective communication with healthcare providers is essential for the successful treatment of depression. Family members can actively participate in this process to ensure the best care for their loved one. Here's how the family can play a role in communicating with healthcare providers:

1. Attending Appointments:

Family members can accompany their loved one to therapy or medical appointments, providing an extra set of ears and offering support during discussions.

2. Taking Notes:

During appointments, family members can take notes on the healthcare provider's recommendations, treatment plans, and any changes to medication or therapy. This helps ensure that nothing is overlooked.

3. Asking Questions:

Family members should feel comfortable asking questions on behalf of their loved one. This can include inquiries about the diagnosis, treatment options, potential side effects, and what to expect in the course of treatment.

4. Sharing Observations:

Family members are in a unique position to observe their loved ones' behaviour and mood on a daily basis. Sharing these observations with healthcare providers can provide valuable insights into the individual's progress or any challenges they are facing.

5. Reporting Side Effects:

If the individual is taking medication, family members should report any observed side effects to the healthcare provider. This information can guide adjustments to the treatment plan.

6. Expressing Concerns:

If the family has concerns about the treatment's effectiveness, side effects, or any other aspect of care, they should not hesitate to express these concerns to the healthcare provider. Open and honest communication is essential.

7. Seeking Clarification:

If there is any confusion or uncertainty about the treatment plan or the nature of depression, family members can seek clarification from the healthcare provider to ensure a clear understanding.

8. Collaborative Decision-Making:

Family members can work collaboratively with healthcare providers in making treatment decisions. This collaborative approach ensures that the treatment plan aligns with the individual's needs and preferences.

9. Advocating for the Individual:

In some situations, the family may need to advocate on behalf of their loved one, especially if the individual is unable to communicate their needs or preferences due to the severity of their depression.

10. Respecting Confidentiality:

While actively participating in their loved one's care, family members should also respect the individual's confidentiality and privacy. It's important to balance involvement while respecting personal boundaries.

3.7 Dealing with CRISIS SITUATIONS

Crisis situations in the context of depression can be challenging, but family members can play a vital role in providing support and ensuring safety.

3.7.1 Alert Signs

Just as the signs for physical health emergencies such as cardiac arrest, choking etc., recognizing the warning signs of a mental health crisis is the first step in effectively responding to a mental health emergency. Talk to your doctor or a psychologist to know what signs can be alarming and how to act to manage the situation. These signs may include:

- **Extreme mood swings:** Rapid and severe shifts in mood, from extreme sadness to extreme irritability or agitation.

- **Isolation:** A sudden withdrawal from social interactions and activities they once enjoyed.

- **Expressions of hopelessness:** Verbalizing feelings of hopelessness, despair, or a lack of purpose.

- **Self-harming or suicidal talk:** Expressing thoughts of self-harm or suicide, even indirectly.

- **Severe anxiety or panic attacks:** Intense and uncontrollable feelings of anxiety or panic.

- **Aggression and attacks:** physical assaults with sharp objects, throwing objects etc.

3.7.2 What to Do in an Emergency?

In the event of a mental health emergency, it's crucial to take immediate action:

Create a safety plan: Collaborate with the person and healthcare providers to make sure that you already have created a safety plan and is in place for managing crisis situations in the future. Include contact information for crisis helplines, supportive individuals, and coping strategies.

Know emergency procedures: Be aware of emergency procedures, and know how to act swiftly in life-threatening situations.

Utilize crisis helplines: Crisis helplines, such as suicide prevention hotlines, are available 24/7. Assist the person in reaching out to these resources for immediate support.

Stay calm: Don't panic. Maintain a calm and non-judgmental demeanour to help de-escalate the situation.

Remove immediate risks: If there's an immediate risk of self-harm or suicide, remove any accessible means that could be used for harm, such as medications or sharp objects.

Contact professionals: Reach out to mental health professionals, crisis hotlines, or emergency services as needed for guidance and immediate help.

Stay with them: Offer to stay with the person during the crisis to provide support and reassurance.

Encourage professional help: If not already involved, encourage the person to seek professional help immediately. Crisis situations often indicate a need for a higher level of care.

Offer reassurance and hope: Remind the person that crises are temporary and that, with help and support, they can overcome the difficulties they are facing.

Safety planning is a critical aspect of managing crisis situations and preventing future emergencies. A safety plan typically includes:

Emergency contacts: A list of crisis hotlines, supportive friends or family members, and healthcare providers to contact during a crisis.

Coping strategies: Techniques and activities that can help the person manage distressing emotions or thoughts.

Triggers and warning signs: Identification of the specific triggers and early warning signs that indicate the potential for a crisis.

Places of safety: Locations where the person can go for support or to escape an unsafe environment during a crisis.

Restricting access: Strategies to limit access to potential means of self-harm or suicide.

Safety planning is a collaborative effort between the individual, their family, and healthcare providers to ensure a proactive and prepared response to crisis situations. It aims to enhance safety, reduce risks, and provide a framework for managing emergencies effectively.

A minute to reflect!

Have you ever had the same attitude towards the medications for mental health issues? Read about the natural mood up lifters? Pick one and do it now, yes! Do it now, before you move on to continue reading!

4. EXTEND LOVE, END STIGMA

(Four E's- pillars of support)

> *"Not every smile has a fairy rose in it, each one has a story, tap the heart to know the fact*
> *To let the voice of the unspoken feelings be heard, Just Listen!" – Dr. Sloka*

You're reading the most important part of the book in the journey of supporting loved ones through the challenges of depression. Depression is not an enemy that someone fights alone. It's a battle that we face together, as families, as friends, as a united front. Let's know how you can be that unwavering source of support without saying but showing them that "I'm here for you" and I'm here with you."

Look at the 4 E's concept on how you can extend love and support, and end the stigma

4.1 E- Empathetic Communication

Empathetic communication is the cornerstone of supporting a loved one through depression. It's not just about the words we use but the compassion and empathy we infuse into every conversation.

When your loved one is experiencing depression, it's essential to remember that their emotions and experiences are valid. They might feel like they're carrying a heavy burden, and your role is not to take that burden away but to help them carry it safely and unload it.

Effective communication with empathy is about listening actively, to hear not just the words but the emotions behind them. Understanding comes from deep listening, being present, allowing the person to share their feelings, not dismissing their thoughts and feelings, and encouraging to seek support.

4.1.1 The Power of Listening

The act of deep listening is the foundation upon which you build trust, empathy, and a resilient bond with your loved one. It is the first step in breaking down the stigma surrounding depression and building human connection.

Listening is a potent and transformative tool in our journey to support loved ones and break down the walls of stigma surrounding depression. It's more than just hearing words; it's about creating a deep connection.

In the realm of depression, where thoughts and feelings can be heavy, listening is like a gentle embrace. It communicates that their experiences and feelings are valid. It's a non-judgmental sanctuary of understanding, a reminder that your loved one is not alone in their struggle.

When you truly listen, you allow the unsaid to surface. You hear the sighs and silences, the emotions that lie beneath the words. Your attention becomes a powerful warm compress that soothes the pain. It tells your loved one that their voice matters, that their pain is acknowledged, and that they are not isolated in their journey.

4.1.2 Effective Conversation Strategies- What to say?

Effective communication is your most powerful ally when supporting a loved one through depression. Here are a few strategies to help you communicate with empathy.

1. **Open-Ended Questions:** Encourage your loved one to share their feelings by asking open-ended questions that go beyond simple "yes" or "no" answers. For example, ask, "How have you been feeling lately?" instead of "Are you feeling better?"

2. **Validate Emotions:** Acknowledge your loved one's emotions and experiences. You can say, "I understand that you're going through a difficult time, and its okay to feel this way" instead of "cheer up dude! Why are so dumb and dull all the time"?

3. **Use "I" Statements:** Express your feelings and concerns using "I" statements. For example, say, "I feel worried when I see you struggling," instead of making accusatory statements.

4. **Offer Reassurance:** Reassure your loved one that you're there for them and that you care. You might say, "I'm here to support you, and we'll get through this together."

5. **Be Patient:** Understand that your loved one may find it difficult to communicate their feelings. Be patient and let them share at their own pace. You could say "I'm here with you, take time to express"

6. **Respect Boundaries:** While it's essential to encourage communication, also respect their boundaries. If they need space, allow them to have it. Don't force them.

7. **Empathize, Don't Minimize:** Avoid minimizing their experiences or offering well-intentioned but dismissive comments like "It's not that tough as compared to what I suffered or faced." Instead, empathize with their feelings, such as "I can see this is really tough for you."

8. **Encourage Professional Help:** Gently suggest seeking professional help, emphasizing that it's a sign of strength to seek assistance from experts. You could use statements like "I'd recommend you to seek a specialist advice", "This needs an expert opinion and shall I help you to find and meet the expert?"

9. **Appreciate:** Acknowledging and appreciating for sharing their feelings make them feel that you valued them trusting you, and also conveys that their concerns are valid and heard. You could say "I'm glad you opened up and shared", "I appreciate you sharing your feelings with me"

4.1.3 Avoiding Common Pitfalls in Communication-what not to say?

While effective communication is crucial when supporting a loved one through depression, it's equally important to avoid common pitfalls that can hinder the process. Here's how to sidestep these traps:

1. **Avoiding Judgment:** Do not judge or criticize your loved one's feelings or experiences. Judgment can make them hesitant to open up. Instead, be empathetic and non-judgmental. Avoid phrases like "you should", "you must", "you have to", "you need to" which make them feel pressured.

2. **Offering Unsolicited Advice:** Refrain from offering solutions or advice unless your loved one explicitly asks for it. Sometimes, they need someone to listen, not provide answers. So, be there with them to pay all you ears. Resist the temptation of offering your own advises.

3. **Minimizing Feelings:** Avoid downplaying their emotions or saying things like "It's not that bad."

Such statements can make them feel misunderstood or unheard. Instead, acknowledge their feelings and struggles.

4. **Comparing Experiences:** Do not compare their situation to your own or someone else's. Each person's experience with depression is unique. Focus on their journey, not yours or others'.

5. **Making It About You:** Resist the urge to turn conversations toward your experiences or problems. While sharing can be helpful, ensure the focus remains on your loved one when they need to talk.

6. **Dismissing Emotions:** Never dismiss or invalidate their feelings. Saying something like "You're overreacting", "hey! That's okay, leave it", "it's time for you to focus on other aspects and enjoy life, not to think this way", "you're educated and mature, didn't expect you thinking this way", "you're focusing much on a trivial thing", can make them feel unheard and unsupported.

7. **Reacting with Frustration:** Understand that your loved one's depression may cause unpredictable emotions or behaviours. Try not to react with frustration or anger. Instead, offer patience and understanding.

8. **Forcing Communication:** If your loved one isn't ready to talk, don't force them. Respect their boundaries and let them know you're there when they're ready to open up.

9. **Ignoring Professional Help:** Encourage seeking professional assistance but don't insist on it. Avoid saying things like "Oh! You don't need therapies or medicines, just follow these remedies and you'll be better soon.", "go on a trip, you'll be fine", "don't take

medicines, they'll have side effects". Instead, offer it as a suggestion and express your support for their decisions.

By avoiding these common communication pitfalls, you create a supportive and safe environment where your loved one can share their feelings and experiences without fear of judgment or criticism. Your words and actions become a source of comfort and understanding, strengthening your connection during their journey to healing.

4.2 E- Emotional Support and Encouragement

Providing emotional support and encouragement means being there for someone in a way that helps them feel understood, cared for, and motivated. It involves offering comfort, empathy, and positive reinforcement, especially during challenging times or when someone is going through difficult situations such as depression. It's about being that constant source of motivation, reminding them that brighter days are definitely possible. But how can you support to instil the hope within them? Read below

1. **Set Realistic Goals:** Help your loved one set achievable goals, no matter how small. These goals create a sense of purpose and direction.

2. **Be Patient:** Understand that healing takes time. Be patient and remind them that it's okay to progress at their own pace.

3. **Create a Vision:** Help them visualize a brighter future. Encourage them to picture the life they want to lead, free from the burdens of depression.

4. **Provide Unconditional Support:** Make it clear that your support is unwavering, regardless of the ups and downs. Your love and encouragement are constant.

5. **Be Their Anchor:** Be a steadfast anchor in the storm of depression. Reassure them that you are here, come what may, and that together, you will weather any challenge.

6. **Remind Them of Progress:** When they face setbacks, remind them of the progress they've already made. Sometimes, it's easy to lose sight of how far they've come.

7. **Offer Affirmations:** Shower them with positive affirmations. Remind them of their strengths, their resilience, and the incredible potential within them.

8. **Celebrate Every Step:** Celebrate every step forward, no matter how small. These celebrations reinforce the idea that progress is happening.

9. **Toolkits:** It is important to streamline the routine schedules, and use of certain tools can be helpful. Plenty of such tools can be found on the internet or you can create a few according to the needs. Tools commonly found helpful include- checklists for routine self-care activities, meal planners, to do lists, medication reminders, medication charts, and day planners, sleep diaries, thought diaries, mood trackers, and gratitude journal. Both paper based and digital tools can be available and the use of technology can make it easier to support the use of these tools.

4.3 E- Engaging

When supporting a loved one dealing with depression, engaging other family members and educating them about depression can be a vital aspect of creating a strong support network.

How to Go About It:

Lead by Example: Be the first to initiate discussions about mental health and share your own experiences or concerns. Leading by example can inspire others to open up.

Choose the Right Time and Place: Pick a comfortable, private, and distraction-free environment for these conversations.

Listen Actively: When a family member speaks about their mental health, listen attentively, without judgment or offering immediate solutions. Sometimes, they just need someone to listen.

Share Resources: Provide information about mental health resources, support groups, and hotlines. Knowledge can empower family members to seek help when needed.

Use Empathetic Language: Choose words and phrases that convey empathy and understanding. Avoid blame, criticism, or stigmatizing language.

Normalize It: Treat conversations about mental health as normal and routine. The more it's discussed, the more normalized it becomes within the family.

Stay Patient: Be patient with family members who might need time to open up. Remember that everyone's journey is unique.

Initiate Conversations: Begin by initiating conversations with other family members about the situation. Share information about depression, its impact, and the importance of support.

Assign Roles: Identify the strengths and capabilities of each family member and assign roles accordingly. For instance, one family member might handle doctor's appointments, while another focuses on emotional support.

Communicate Openly: Encourage open and honest communication among family members. Everyone should feel comfortable sharing their concerns, ideas, and feelings.

Educate Everyone: Ensure that everyone in the family has a basic understanding of depression, its symptoms, and how it can be managed. Knowledge empowers individuals to provide better support.

Respect Individual Boundaries: While involving other family members, respect their boundaries and personal limitations. Not everyone may be able to contribute in the same way, and that's okay.

Hold Regular Family Meetings: Set up regular family meetings to discuss the individual's progress, share insights, and address any challenges or concerns.

Provide Support for Each Other: Remember that supporting someone with depression can be emotionally taxing. Make sure that family members are also taking care of themselves and seeking support when needed.

Celebrate Small Victories: Celebrate the progress and victories, no matter how small. It reinforces the idea that the family is working together to support their loved one.

Join Campaigns: Look for local and national mental health campaigns that resonate with you. These may include awareness walks, fundraising events, or social media campaigns. Involve family members to join these campaigns and programs.

Encourage Participation: Encourage your friends and family to join campaigns as well. The more people involved, the greater the impact.

Leverage Your Skills: Use your unique skills or talents to contribute to campaigns. Whether you're good at organizing events or creating compelling content, your skills can be invaluable.

Involving other family members is a collaborative effort that not only lightens the load on one individual but also strengthens the overall support system. It ensures that the person with depression receives well-rounded care and emotional support from their entire family, fostering a more positive and hopeful environment for everyone involved.

4.4 E- Educate family and beyond

Educating your family members about depression is a crucial step in creating a supportive environment for your loved one. Some tips on how to do it effectively:

How to Educate Family Members:

Provide Information: Share educational resources, such as articles, books, or documentaries about depression. Point them to reputable sources of information such as helplines, local mental health services, support groups.

Lead Discussions: Initiate family discussions about depression. Encourage questions and offer explanations.

Use Relatable Language: Explain concepts in simple and relatable terms. Avoid using overly technical or clinical language that may be confusing.

Share Personal Experiences: If you or your loved one with depression is comfortable, share personal experiences with the condition. Real-life stories can make the information more relatable.

Attend Workshops or Support Groups: Consider attending workshops or support groups together as a family. Hearing from experts or others with similar experiences can be enlightening.

Correct Misconceptions: Address any misconceptions or myths about depression that may arise. Provide accurate information to dispel misunderstandings.

Encourage Questions: Let family members know that it's okay to ask questions and seek clarification. Create an open and non-judgmental atmosphere for discussions. Ask open ended questions.

Reiterate the Importance of Support: Emphasize the role of family support in the recovery process. Explain that the family's understanding and assistance are essential.

These are some of the ways that can help break down the stigma, promote understanding about mental health and also builds a supportive family culture.

ENCOURAGING OPEN CONVERSATIONS BEYOND THE FAMILY

Opening up conversations about mental health beyond the family circle can have a profound impact on reducing stigma and fostering understanding. Here's how to do it in a friendly and motivational way:

Start Small: You don't need to launch a big campaign; small steps matter. Begin by discussing mental health with close friends or colleagues. Share your experiences, if you're comfortable, and encourage them to do the same.

Normalize Conversations: In your interactions, normalize discussions about mental health. Treat it like any other topic. By doing this, you show that it's okay to talk about it.

Active Listening: When someone opens up about their mental health, be an active listener. Offer your full attention, ask questions, and validate their feelings. This creates a safe space for sharing.

Use social media: Social media platforms are excellent for reaching a broader audience. Share informative posts, personal stories, or articles related to mental health. Your posts can inspire others to join the conversation.

Organize Informal Gatherings: discuss mental health in a relaxed setting. Create an environment where they feel safe sharing their thoughts.

Invite Experts: Consider inviting mental health experts or advocates to speak at local events or webinars. Their knowledge and experience can provide valuable insights to the community.

Share Resources: Point people to useful resources, such as websites, helplines, or support groups. Let them know where they can find more information or seek help if needed.

Be a Role Model: By initiating these conversations and being open about mental health, you set an example for others. Your willingness to discuss it encourages them to do the same.

Keep the Momentum: Consistency is the key. Keep on the momentum going by regularly discussing around mental health and well-being. The more it's talked about, the more it becomes a natural part of our conversations.

Encouraging open conversations beyond the family is a powerful way to break down the barriers of stigma. Your friendly and motivational approach can inspire others to embrace the dialogue around mental health, seek support when needed, and ultimately create a more empathetic and understanding community.

A minute to reflect!

Think of a time when your friend or a family member was sharing their feelings with you and you had either reacted or responded. Broadened your perspective around the active listening now? Talk to someone, check on their well-being and as they share, just listen actively! Look at how much difference does it make in their day

5. RECOVERY

> *"Remember! The suffering isn't anymore a constant, the recovery isn't any instant"* – Dr. Sloka

Recovery is the beating heart of this section, reminding us that healing is not just a concept but a tangible reality. It's about rediscovering one's self, reclaiming a sense of purpose, and rebuilding the foundations of a fulfilling life. It's proof that, even in the most challenging times, the human spirit can regenerate, like a phoenix rising from its ashes.

If you're suffering or you ever suffered depression, as you delve into this chapter, let it be a reminder that no journey is in vain. Every step you've taken, every word you've read, and every action you've contemplated has brought you to this point—a point where hope shines brightly, where recovery is within reach, and where reflection unveils the wisdom born from the journey. In these pages, you'll find the inspiration to move forward, the strength to embrace recovery, and the wisdom to reflect on the path you've walked.

5.1 The Real Story of Hope and Resilience

Here is a beautiful and inspiring story of a young man who battled depression and found hope and resilience with the support of their loved ones:

A Young man, a medical professional in India, proactive and highly enthusiastic, with many aspirations landed in his dream country, the UK for his higher studies but the reality wasn't as fanciful as he imagined with everything being new to adjust- the place, people, culture, education system, currency and part time job. Adjustment has become an issue.

It was during one fateful ice-skating adventure that his life took an unexpected, chilling turn. As he stepped onto the ice, a few minutes of skating led to a bone-chilling fall, followed by a gut-wrenching cracking sound. Fear and terror surged through him, and he was swiftly moved away to the accident and emergency unit where the news was grim: a nasty fracture, they said, demanding urgent surgery.

He was shattered and broken, he cried in despair, his mind awash with worries about his studies, finances to manage bills and expenses, and the deep longing for the warmth and support of his faraway parents. It was as if life had reached a dead end.

He was taken into the operation theatre and after a few hours of sleep to anaesthesia, slowly tried to open eyes but leg was feeling heavy and unable to move, could hear nurse whispering "surgery successful".

The Discharge notes revealed the extent of damage- a metallic road and seven nails held his leg together. Back at home, bed ridden, gloomy all time, no hope on anything, feelings of "why only me" covered him in darkness, home sick, guilt of going to ice skating, and suffered the depression. Appetite changed, lost weight, muscle wasting occurred, nutritional deficiencies set in. He used to sleep hungry at times, he needed to take 4 tablets 4 times a day for pain relief and injections to prevent blood clots. The pain of injections everyday was another terrible struggle to live with. It was an absolute hard task to get off the stairs at house to get into ambulance every time he needed to visit the hospital for managing follow up appointments in the extreme cold weather. His leg had multiple staples to be removed and the pain while removal of staples and bleeding was at the top of his throat and being alone far away from the family during the crisis was another excruciating emotional burden adding to the physical pain.

With passing days, slowly pain in the leg started to ease with regular medications, flat mates stepped in with good support, preparing meals, packed in boxes at each time of the meal, sitting with him sometimes and talk to distract and support.

Few other friends used to ring up and say everything is going to be okay, not to feel bad as got everyone to support in terms of food. But suffering is personal and others could not understand. Several days passed without even seeing the sunlight. Un-empathetic words from people although depressing, made stronger, as he realized he was responsible for his own life and recovery and peace of mind.

He realized he cannot control the situation but he can surely do his best to utilize the housebound time as a phase of rest and make it productive. He decided to start focusing on academic work, arranged virtual meetings with tutors, made a plan, established a routine- used to work on assignments, eat food, take medicines regularly, attend appointments, exercise regularly, connect with family, watch any series or movies, talk to friends and sleep early.

After a few days, he was advised to walk on braces and so he informed that he wanted to re-join the work, so his manager supported with flexible working hours, colleagues were cooperative by not assigning any work that involved walking, regularly checking on him, one friend supported his travel to work place by dropping and picking up. Also, the director of his course at the university used to attend him in person to check on him regularly and offered support.

After a month, he took a flight back home where he found good care and support by the family. As this was going on well, his depression has set back with stereotypical comments passed by a physiotherapist when she used the phrases- "a boy is expected to be strong enough, you lack muscle, you must go to gym to build muscle, a boy is expected to have good muscle". He lost hopes in recovery and felt it is going to be a permanent disability and cannot walk properly at all.

But upon advice and support from the family, visited another physiotherapist who advised exercises, offered reassurance. His mother had been a constant source of support who encouraged him to do exercises regularly and he was able to walk much better and moved back to the UK soon to finish his studies.

With unyielding determination, he threw himself into his academics, maintained regular contact with his tutors, and even managed to complete his dissertation on time. The result was nothing short of remarkable: a distinction and he was the only student from the whole of his batch to graduate despite the physical and mental challenges and also bagged the prestigious honour -the university's best academic award.

It was a proud moment for him to celebrate after a long battle with depression and physical health challenges.

The journey wasn't over by then and not without any setbacks. When she shares his feelings with his friends, he finds it depressing to hear phrases like "you're matured and not to think this way", "you're over thinking", "just leave it, don't focus much on it", "and enjoy the time". But he felt that all those comments made him stronger and are probably the reason for this book to be brought out.

It means, by now, you must have understood whose story you've been reading!

5.2 The Reflection

So, what must have happened during the journey that made him suffer depression and was able to overcome? The reflection on the story is quite insightful and offers a comprehensive understanding of the various factors that played a role in the man's journey from depression to recovery. Those factors were:

1. **Predisposing factors**: The man's pre-existing adjustment issues with his new environment set the stage for his vulnerability to depression.

2. **Precipitating factors**: The traumatic incident of the ice-skating fall acted as a significant trigger that precipitated his depression. It emphasizes how unexpected events can exacerbate mental health challenges.

3. **Aggravating factors**: Nutritional deficiencies and the struggle to manage his daily needs worsened his overall health. This factor underscores the importance of addressing both physical and mental health needs in recovery.

4. **Triggering factors**: Negative comments and dismissive attitudes from friends added to his emotional burden. These remarks acted as triggers that perpetuated his depression, highlighting the impact of the social environment on mental health.

Recovery factors: The story illustrates that the journey to recovery was made possible through several factors:

1. **Support from friends and family**: Their support and encouragement played a pivotal role in his recovery. It

emphasizes the importance of having a strong support system during challenging times.

2. **Positive outlook**: The man's determination to focus on academics and career goals demonstrates the power of a positive mind-set. This positive outlook can act as a driving force for recovery.

3. **Adherence to treatment and exercises**: Following medical advice and rehabilitation exercises was crucial for his physical recovery. It emphasizes the importance of adhering to prescribed treatments in mental and physical health recovery.

4. **Nutritional support**: Addressing nutritional deficiencies was vital for his overall well-being. It highlights the connection between nutrition and mental health.

5. **Use of checklists and to-do lists**: Organizing daily activities with checklists and to-do lists helped him regain a sense of control and structure in his life. This technique can be a valuable tool for individuals dealing with depression or anxiety.

6. **Taking breaks and self-care**: Watching movies and taking breaks helped him recharge and find moments of solace. Self-care is essential for maintaining mental well-being.

In summary, the reflection highlights how a combination of factors, both positive and negative, influenced the young man's journey from depression to recovery.

5.3 Navigating Setbacks and Challenges

Navigating setbacks and challenges in the form of relapses and recurrences through the journey of battling depression can be difficult, but it's an essential part of the recovery process. Here's how to do it:

1. Acceptance:

Understand that setbacks are a normal part of the journey. Depression recovery is not always a linear process, and occasional relapses or challenges are common.

2. Identify triggers:

Knowing what triggers low mood can help recognise the depressive episodes and help deal with it safely

3. Self-Compassion:

Be kind and compassionate toward yourself. Understand that setbacks don't define your progress or worth. Treat yourself with the same care you'd offer a loved one.

4. Seek Support:

Lean on your support system, including friends, family, or a mental health professional. Share your challenges and seek guidance. You don't have to go through it alone.

5. Revaluate Goals:

If necessary, reassess your goals and expectations. Adjust them to be more realistic and achievable, especially during challenging times.

6. Self-Care:

Prioritize self-care. Focus on getting enough rest, maintaining a healthy diet, and engaging in physical activity. These actions can help you better cope with challenges.

7. Mindfulness and Coping Strategies:

Practice mindfulness and coping strategies you've learned during your recovery journey. These tools can help you manage setbacks effectively.

8. Professional Guidance:

If the challenges persist or become overwhelming, consider seeking additional or more intensive professional help. Therapy or medication adjustments may be necessary.

9. Learn from Setbacks:

Use setbacks as opportunities for learning and growth. Identify what triggered the setback and develop strategies to avoid or manage those triggers in the future.

Remember that overcoming setbacks and challenges is a testament to your resilience. With the right support and coping strategies, you can continue to make progress in your battle with depression.

5.4 A Future Filled with Hope

A future filled with hope is a radiant dawn after the darkest night. It's the belief that no matter how deep the struggles are, there's always a path to light and happiness. In the journey of overcoming depression, this hopeful future is not a distant dream; it's a reality waiting to be embraced.

With each step forward, you're crafting a future where joy, peace, and fulfilment flourish. It's a future where laughter rings louder than despair, where your dreams shine brighter than doubts, and where every sunrise promises new opportunities for happiness.

The battles you've fought, the resilience you've shown, and the support of loved ones have paved the way to this hopeful horizon. It's a future where your experiences with depression become a source of strength, wisdom, and empathy, not a chain that holds you back.

In this hopeful future, you're not merely surviving; you're thriving. You're writing a story of triumph over adversity, and your journey is an inspiration to others. It's a future where you cherish the small victories, acknowledge your progress, and find purpose in helping others on their own paths to recovery.

FINAL WORDS

In a single line, "**Not Just Sadness; the silence needs to be heard**" is more than a book; it's a guide to a transformative journey. I can't believe if we reached the end of this journey but yes, we've covered the depths of depression, the shadow of stigma, and the power of love and understanding. We've delved into the challenges, celebrated the victories, and embraced the hope that radiates from personal growth.

Our journey through this book has made one thing clear: depression does not define a person, nor does it define a family. Instead, it is an obstacle that, with the right support and approach, can be overcome. Families play a pivotal role in this process, standing alongside their loved ones through the highs and lows and all families together make a society. If families can transform into non-stigmatizing, non-stereotypical systems, all then we can find is the society with a stronger mental health.

Remember! You never know the storm behind the smiles in the other person, so watch your words before you speak; they need not offer comfort, if at least not add any weight to the already ongoing struggle.

Thank you for your time, and patience in reading this book until here. Your role in breaking the stigma is pivotal, and your love is a powerful force for healing.

As I conclude, what I wish for? You just read and close the book? No!

May this book become a source of guidance for those facing the complexities of depression! May it encourage open conversations, understanding, and the breaking down of the walls of stigma! May it empower families to be the support systems that their loved ones need. Do you have someone on your mind who you'd think needs to read this book? Gift them a copy ☺

Dr. Sloka

REFERENCES

Antipsychotics | Royal College of Psychiatrists

Bains, N., & Abdijadid, S. (2023). Major Depressive Disorder. In StatPearls. StatPearls Publishing.

Bhatia, R. (2023) *What is psychotherapy? Psychiatry.org - What is Psychotherapy?* Available at: https://www.psychiatry.org/patientsfamilies/psychotherapy (Accessed: October 2023)

Biological, Psychological, and Social Determinants of Depression: A Review of Recent Literature—PMC.

Chand, S. P., & Arif, H. (2023). Depression. In StatPearls. StatPearls Publishing.

Depression—An overview | ScienceDirect Topics.

Gander, F., Proyer, R. T., Ruch, W., & Wyss, T. (2013). Strength-based positive interventions: Further evidence for their potential in enhancing well-being and alleviating depression. Journal of Happiness Studies, 14(4), 1241-1259.

Myths and Facts About Depression | Psych Central.

National Research Council (US) and Institute of Medicine (US) Committee on Depression, P. P., England, M. J., & Sim, L. J. (2009). The Etiology of Depression. In Depression in Parents, Parenting, and Children: Opportunities to Improve Identification, Treatment, and Prevention. National Academies Press (US).

NIMH » Depression

Non-Medical Prescribing NICE. Available at: https://bnf.nice.org.uk/medicines-guidance/non-medical prescribing/

Protected characteristics | Equality and Human Rights Commission

Psychiatry.org—Stigma, Prejudice and Discrimination Against People with Mental Illness.

Six common depression types (2017, January 23) Harvard Health

Stigma: A Unique Source of Distress for Family Members of Individuals with Mental Illness—PMC.

Suicide Warning Signs: What to Look Out For.

Symptoms—Depression in adults (2021, February 15) Nhs.Uk

The 5 Fundamental Differences Between Sadness and Depression.

Varma, S. *Peripartum Depression (formerly postpartum), Psychiatry.org - Peripartum Depression (formerly Postpartum)*. Available at: https://www.psychiatry.org/patients-families/postpartum-depression

Not Just Sadness

The silence needs to be heard!

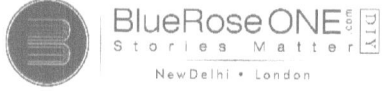

NewDelhi • London

www.ingramcontent.com/pod-product-compliance
Ingram Content Group UK Ltd.
Pitfield, Milton Keynes, MK11 3LW, UK
UKHW041944230426
12048UKWH00008B/131